Danielle Chevalier

MY TRICK
FOR LOSING WEIGHT
WITHOUT
DIETING

Edition SIP – Monaco

CONTENTS

FIRST PART: SLIM IN PEACE

SECOND PART: LIVE IN PEACE
WITH YOURSELF

THIRD PART:
LIGHT FAMILY RECIPES TO HELP YOU SLIM

PREFACE

TO BE READ FIRST

What is my trick for losing weight without dieting?

It is very simple, so simple that you will have trouble believing in it. Yet it works. It has worked for me. It has worked for all my friends who wanted to lose weight, and since I revealed my trick in the present book, I keep receiving letters of thanks by the hundreds.

This is my trick in all its incredible simplicity: Eat much, much, much slower than usual. To do this, you only need to learn to chew your food for a long, a very long time (see pages 60, 70, 77 to 82, 94, 150).

Now you probably do not believe this. Neither did I! But since I had nothing to lose, I tried it. The result? Loss of 6 and a half pounds in the first week. Loss of 13 pounds in the following weeks. Altogether 19 and a half pounds.

The results obtained by all my friends have been just as spectacular.

You may choose not to believe in it; but at least try it for 3 days and then weigh yourself!

You will be very, very pleasantly surprised.

In this book, I will tell you how to eat easily MUCH, *much more slowly.*

I, who have tried everything in order to lose weight, will also tell you how to obtain the desired results faster. Once more, if you eat very slowly and if you know how to chew your food thoroughly, this is enough for you to lose weight, just as I did. But you will also find many other things in this book.

I therefore advise you to read it: not only will you lose weight even faster, while enhancing your looks, *but you will also discover in it a real health-investment.*

Read on and see for yourself.

FOREWORD

In this book you won't find any dull scientific explanations, except for those required in order to clarify our point of view.

You also won't find any diagrams, scientific statistics nor any complicated or cruelly restrictive diets in it.

We will not talk about subtile techniques or psychic conditioning which require the support of a specialist. For that purpose there are specialised institutes and we surely don't want to intrude into their field.

NO.

What you will find here, is first of all COMPREHENSION.

Even if, on first thought, it might seem rather common, we are very interested in your daily life with its environments and its limits. In all this we will try to picture your personality, your problems and your possibilities.

Must you slim? Can you achieve this without causing confusion in your daily life? Are you yourself capable of finding the necessary moral and physical balance that you'll need? This approach of your-self is our STARTING-POINT.

Further on you'll find some friendly advice, a few simple, but well tested, methods - precautions to take, traps to avoid, basic principles to assimilate. All this clearly expressed. It's more like an everyday conversation, a friendly chat.

11

Yet we are sure that this book could become very important to you, firstly because of the numerous practical suggestions concerning family, household and cooking and secondly of the moral support you'll find in it, which will come in useful in all circumstances.

A simple, clear, useful book (at least we hope so), but in any case, a very enjoyable one to read.

FIRST PART
SLIM IN PEACE

CHAPTER I

WAYS AND SYSTEMS

Methods, ways, measurements, massages, SLIMMING.

Theory, techniques, tactics, treatments, Waist Measurements.

Fat, calories, chemistry, vitamins, DIETS - DIETS. — Ah, there we are, the key-word for all this huge variety that is available to us in order to reduce, diminish, vanish, all this extra fat that bothers us, tires us, makes us ugly and last but not least scares us, for it is said that it is UNHEALTHY for us and quickens our end!

Diets? Surely, for the last 20 years or more we have been introduced to all kinds of them, from the craziest up to the most scientific. But in the course of time only a few of them have proved to give enough satisfactory and proportionally durable results as to claim: « Ah, finally, Here it is, the right way to nourish, to stay slender, supple and healthy. That's what we must do, not only to lose weight, but to achieve and maintain a good, normal balance: « Height/ Weight without privations, without slackness, without continuous restrictions.

Surely, where is the benefit of losing 10, 20, or even 50 pounds, if it leaves us exhausted, weak, sad for evermore, in front of our dishes composed of steamed carrots and hard boiled eggs!, or if by the slightest excess, pounds come back? What if your enjoyment of life doesn't return with regained slimness?

Surely, while adding together several systems, psychological modification by revolutionary methods, extreme rules of living, sports, severely controlled nourishment, numerous people have obtained good results.

But at what price? With what effort?, what strain and never ending surveillance!... And, with the permanent and indispensable help of dieticians, of specialists, of severe and vigilant supervisors, always there to minimise discouragement, and revolt!

For not everybody has this infallible will, required for a radical and lasting change of nourishment and way of life.

If you think you have this strengtht of mind, or, if you have the possibility of being helped, supervised, supported in your efforts for losing weight in a durable and progressive way, you can try it and we wish you Good-Luck!

But what if you are alone with your problem, if a demanding, or simply indifferent, family forces you to eat « just like everybody else », if you are far away from any sport center, if you can't afford regular consultations from a specialist or to be a regular guest at an expensive « health farm? »

Must you therefore keep your rolls of fat, your heavy legs, your rotund belly?

Must you stay there with nothing else to do but sigh and dream of the time you were slim and alert?, hide yourself, shapelessly dressed in wide dull clothing? Renounce the joys of the open air, swimming in the sea, dancing? Suffer from complexes and jealousy?

NO.

Don't remain in your solitude with your regrets. Remember that the human body — Yours — is made to stay in a balance of fat and muscles, until the end. That the excessive formation of fat is a MISTAKE, not a final catastrophy, and that every mistake can be corrected if one wants to.

Now you know you're not alone anymore and that you are to take « yourself » under control, while relying on some simple basics and some friendly, but sensible, advice.

It will be like a spring cleaning, weeding a garden corner, a dress altered, a motor repaired, a room redecorated.

Those jobs, surely you've done some of them already? It didn't seem impossible to you did it? So then, why not start an entire renovation of your body?

It's not more difficult, believe us.

All it takes is decision, gathering the necessary tools and ingredients and starting.

First of all it is imperative to make up a BALANCE with no indulgence but also without extreme rigidness.

We have known young women, very slim, who were obsessed by 2 extra inches on their waist or by having difficulties squeezing their hips into a pair of trousers they wore before pregnancy.

We also see really obese people squeezing themselves into clothing obviously too small and then claim: « they are a size 42! ».

Others mock openly those who seem to be heavier than they are and so are satisfied by visual differences only.

To those 2 categories of people we can't offer anything, unless, from now on, they become concious of reality.

NO, we wrote this book for you, who are lucid, reasonable and know yourselves.

CHAPTER II

WHAT TO THINK OF THE RELATION BETWEEN «HEIGHT – WEIGHT»

Diagrams concerning relations between «Height-Weight» have been drawn by all specialists dealing with treatments and diets for slimming.

And it's filled with anguish those who consult them in order to hear the verdict: « How Many Superfluous pounds ». But all those diagrams, or at least the dozen we have chosen to examine, among all those published, were revealed to be DIFFERENT!

For instance, a German doctor will allow you 120 pounds for a height of 5 foot 3, where an American dietician will grant you 130 pounds for the same height, but a French institute will cruelly bring your weight down to 110 pounds!

Measurements of waist, hips, and buttocks are all different. Well then, who is to be believed?

The best thing to do is to bear in mind that a SATISFACTORY weight is the one we had when we were feeling happy, light, supple and when we had ENDURANCE.

Sir, at the age of 28, your weight was 150 pounds for a height of 5 foot 6, were you in good shape then?

Madam, when you were 23 years old you weighed 120 pounds for a height of 5 foot 3 and everybody thought of you as being ravishing, because you looked so alive and happy?

Well then, why not be satisfied by regaining the weight you had then, adding some 5 or 6 pounds that are granted to you to compensate for the extra years, and don't bother anymore about statistics and diagrams.

«But then», you'll ask us «how many superfluous pounds does it take before we can speak of obesity? »

This is our answer:

« Starting from the first pound, that really bothers you, makes you feel heavy, deforms you, forces you to alter or widen your clothes, give up a sport, dancing, high heels ».

It can happen at the third or only at the twentieth extra pound that you will become aware of that uncomfortable feeling, a feeling that depresses you and finally make you exclaim: « That's enough! » — It HAS TO STOP!

But there again it's YOUR game and YOU are controlling it. Not your scale nor your tape measure. It is your eyes, your body itself, you « Yourself » that will react to the alarming symptoms.

From the moment the alarm goes off you must react. But there again, it's up to YOU to turn off the alarm.

We don't want to give a lecture on the different origins of obesity. When it's pathologic it's up to the physician, especially the endocrinologist to interfere. Surely it will be his treatment that will be the most important. The way of living, of nourishing, will be nothing more than an addition to his prescribed treatment. It will be to only that extent that the person whom it concerns will be able to complete and especially maintain the results obtained by hormonal therapy by himself.

Whatever may be the cause — or causes — of your obesity, and on condition of course that it's real and not imaginary, what will follow must interest you and help you.

24

CHAPTER III

YOUR IDEAL SHAPE

First of all, while you « Have to » be ambitious about the obtained results don't go imagining yourself resembling some cover-girl by next month.

You will always stay « YOU » with your thighs just one inch too short, or with your sloping, shoulders, or with your tiny breasts. But then, even mannequins or models aren't spared from imperfections of physical beauty. THEY, have the photographer's genius to diminish them or cover them up. In fact, the thing that counts most, is « GENERAL AP-PEARANCE », and most of all the fact that you must be « FEELING GOOD ».

So, you will stay « YOUR OWN SELF » but more sup-ple, more resistant, and estheticaly closer to that ideal shape you rediscovered in your memories. In order to always bear in mind this ideal shape you want to see again in your mirror, try to find one of those full-length pictures of yourself you're so proud of.

You must have, hidden somewhere, in your files, a pic-ture you look at with nostalgia, a picture showing you in a bathing-suit, with a slim waist and gently muscled thighs. Or maybe your wedding picture, where your figure seems so fragile. Have it enlarged and hung up in your bath-room or your kitchen. So what, if it makes the others smile!

This MODEL is there for the sole purpose of encoura-ging you.

It will be as if, each time you look at it, the person in the picture is telling you secretly: « In Fact You Are Still ». Like This. This is The Real You. All it takes is a little shaking off of this fat. Beneath it you will find a healthy skin.

In fact this MODEL must be YOU and not one of those stars nor a high-class mannequin.

So then, is the picture ready? It is hung up:

Then we can proceed.

CHAPTER IV

HOW DOES
FAT ACCUMULATE

There is no use in hiding the truth. Everybody agrees by saying that 90% of all obese are those people who either eat too much or eat the wrong things. Reasons for these excesses, or errors, are complex, and different: we can even state that every one of us constitutes a different « case ».

That's why, in each problem concerning overweight it is up to each individual to study and observe himself. This is not to be considered as egoism or indulgence. WE MUST BE INTERESTED IN OURSELVES if we want to achieve amelioration and at the same time feel good.

In order to know if you eat too much or wrongly, and therefore, be able to cope with those excesses or errors, it is imperative to draw up an inventory of whatever you eat daily. Take a note-book and write down all you eat during the day and do this for a whole week. Don't forget anything and make sure you write down when you take your meals or those little in between snacks. Yes, even the grape-fruit you had at 4p.m. or the bar of chocolate you nibbled watching T.V. or the spoonfuls of stew you tasted in order to make sure it's spicy enough.

Here follows an example, given to us by a person who, since then, has progressively changed her body and has regained the joy of living.

Scrupulously, she had written down EVERYTHING she had eaten daily and did this for a whole week. Of course we had to summarise those daily notes, omitting alimentary details and we obtained the following results of an ordinary day: This is what it came down to:

— 7a.m.: one cup of coffee with two lumps of sugar.

— 8a.m.: One cup of coffee, milk and two lumps of sugar, a buttered sandwich with marmalade or two pieces of toast with honey.

— 10.30a.m.: one biscuit (my stomach aches!).

— 12a.m.: a meal taken together with the children: first course: Raw vegetables with hard boiled eggs or paté - meat or fish, with noodles or chips - cheese (camembert or roquefort), - fruit - one glass of wine - three slices of bread - and especially for me: coffee with sugar.

— 3.30p.m.: tea or coffee with cake or biscuits (if a friend drops by to visit, or with the children).

— 8p.m.: together with my husband and children: vegetable soup with butter or cream - potato stew and bacon - or ham - or scrambled eggs or grilled sausages with appropriate dressing (mashed potatoes - canned baby peas - vegetable au « gratin ») - youghourt - pie or custard - two or three slices of bread.

— 10p.m.: one infusion with two lumps of sugar (one glass of water about two o'clock in the morning).

We haven't taken into account occasional additions such as cocktails, salted biscuits, that one has when receiving friends. In our country it reveals bad manners if you don't offer a drink to your guests. So a cocktail or a small Scotch is a must ».

This example shows clearly what a French family generally eats, some differences allowed where it concerns meat and dessert.

This is on condition, of course, that the housewife finds the time to do a little cooking: soups - stews - pies.

We add to those menus some raw-vegetables (tomatoes - salads) some fruit (for vitamins) - some yoghourt (for the children's digestion) and so we think we have given all the necessary ingredients to our family to keep them healthy.

It is true that in this nourishment all necessary ingredients are present for survival, for energy and for growth: fats - proteins - sugars - vitamins - nothing is omitted.

Nevertheless, if, with this nourishment, children are in good shape and « grow up » well, the adults don't seem to be feeling so happy; they suffer from oppressiveness, a decline of their vitality, intestinal gases and slowly, but surely they watch their stomachs grow heavy, their hips widen, their legs lose their mobility.

This is all understandable. A child uses a lot of energy for its growth and, a few exceptions omitted , doesn't pile up extra fat in its tissues.

Beside, his daily activities are very important (running - games - sports - school work) in accordance with his size, and so he has no problems dealing with his calories.

In contrast, the adult, even if very active, doesn't need to grow extra bone and if he eats the same and as much as a child, he will inevitably find himself with an extra dose of « combustible » (energy).

It is clear that this extra « combustible », provided mostly from sugars and starches will, as a result of a chemical process, turn into fat. This fat that little by little surrounds our muscles and organs, will cause psychological troubles such a WEARINESS - HEAVINESS - SWELLING - SHORTNESS OF BREATH - A FATAL SLOWING DOWN OF ALL ACTIVITIES.

By a complex, but logical, follow-up (succession), all this will unbalance your metabolic system, that on a nutritional level, will result in insufficiency concerning needs and defences of the organism. Vicious circle. Hunger remains (it may even increase) but the organism can't transform all this food into energy anymore, no more than it can transform the oxygen of the air we breath.

Those wastes, and extras will be stacked away as fat in the fatty tissue and they won't be disposed of anymore. They Are There To Stay. And soon, as happened to the lady we talked about before, the Twentieth Extra Pound will appear. The scale accuses, for the dressmaker it's a fact, discreetly the children will start making remarks about Mummy turning into « La Mamma » or their Daddy into a « fatty » ...it starts a real panic.

So, we skip a meal - grab our bike or immediately start a series of exhausting floor exercises, we swallow diurétics or one of those « appetite-losers » in order to fill our stomach a quarter of an hour before meals.

By these rather harsh methods we can surely lose, and quickly, two or three pounds, but even so we quickly start feeling empty and exhausted. The heartbeat becomes iregular, we feel sick in the morning, lose our vitality, have a stomach ache, and our intestines become lazy.

To cut things short, by the end of two weeks we would gladly sell our souls to get a doughnut or sausages and chips.

Is this the right solution? No, then what are we to do?

CHAPTER V

THE EXPERIMENTS
WE ARE NOT TO DO

In order to divert your mind we have written down several anecdotes, or should we say conversations, we overheard in different places. They really show us how helpless people can become when they try to get rid of their extra fat.
— Madam A (at the chemists): Give me another package of that herb extract X. I think it does me a great deal of good.

— The chemist: Have you already taken your second dose? How many times a day do you drink this extract? You know that in order to stimulate the kidneys and to obtain a good fluid elimination, it takes only one cup before bedtime.

— Madam A: Yes, yes, I know, but I had no result whatsoever so now I take it also in the morning and during the daytime. I must go to the toilet very often and I'm sure I'm going to lose weight.

— Chemist: In order to lose weight I would rather advise you to watch what you are eating, because if you take too many diuretics you will disorganise your kidneys and lose too much mineral salts.

— Madame A: How can that be?

— Chemist: An overdose of diuretics eliminates the phosphorus and all the mineral salts we need. We must not have too many of them.

— A client: They told me this incredible trick to slim. You only eat one thing a day.

— Madam A: Really!

— The client: Yes, one day roasted rabbit, one day oranges, one day French beans, one day nothing but minced meat. It seems you lose 2 pounds a week.

— Chemist: Yes, and one certainly loses ones mind too on such a diet. Just you try to feed your family is such a way, you will see how happy they will be.

— Madam A: I'll have a revolution going on witihin three days. I prefer my herb infusion.

— Chemist: Yes, but make sure not to overdo it and don't have any illusions. You won't get rid of your fat this way!

Another story

— Madam B: (at a school reunion): It lasts too long. I have such a headache.

— The lady next to her: Have a tablet or go into the fresh air.

— Madam B: I don't know why I'm having these headaches. I never had them before. It must be my liver, undoubtedly. Although, with my diet, my liver shouldn't be causing any trouble.

— Neighbour: Ah, you're on a diet? Without being indiscreet, is it for your liver?

— Madam B: No, I gained weight, this last time. At least 20 pounds, in a couple of months. So I fasted. I was advised by a friend of mine.

— Neighbour: Fasted? COMPLETELY?

— Madam B: Yes, almost nothing, only One pint of water and one apple a day. She followed this diet while being in a German hospital, it seems to give results quickly. Afterwards you can start eating almost normally.

— Neighbour: How long have you been doing this?

— Madam B: It will be Four days now. But it's very hard.

— Neighbour: No wonder you have headaches. I even ask myself how you can still stand up.

I think you'd better start nourishing yourself normally, without delay. What about your Physician?

— Madame B: Oh, he doesn't know anything about it. He would surely forbid me to go on with it.

— Neighbour: You're not reasonable. I don't want to lecture you, but if I were you I would start right away, tonight, by eating some soup and some compote for instance, and from tomorrow on I would have some more solid food. Otherwise you will become seriously ill. No wonder your friend was under the doctors care. You can't do this on your own.

— Madam B: Yes, but then what am I to do?

— Neighbour: I've already told you: be sensible. Diminish, but don't Abolish. One or even two days of fasting won't do any harm, but if you keep it up can become very dangerous. Believe me!

Yes, the chemist in the first story and the neighbour in the second story were both RIGHT.

« To exaggerate in anything, is always wrong » the proverb says, but even more so where or if your HEALTH is concerned. Because here it really concerns the health of these people, who are using « miracle methods » for slimming in a very irresponsible way.

And, we don't even mention, the total abolition of salt or sugar, the products to cut down appetite such as laxatives, iodine etc...

All this is as futile and dangerous as the glasses of vinegar young women used to drink and which caused many intestinal-and stomach troubles.

All this can be tried out eventually, but with extreme precautions and under permanent medical supervision.

So, all this is to be banished from our book, as our only purpose is to help you to diminish your extra fat in a gentle way, without traumas, either for you or for your relatives, but by iust « EATING WELL ».

In fact, we don't have the intention of proposing to you a new miracle diet. There are so many of them already Even so some of them are very good and have proved to be a success for a great many people who were able to follow them in a strict and scrupulous way. But generally, those diets proved to be very difficult to adapt into feeding a Family. It's not only batchelors who want to lose weight. Father, mothers of a family, relatives living with them, adolescents, they all can have weight problems. Is this a sufficient reason to feed everybody with yoghurts and saltless biscuits? And what is more, these diets frequently require articles that are difficult to find or are rather expensive.

Not everybody has the possibility to easily find soya shoots, fresh salmon or full rice. So, most of us must adapt to a way of nourishment thats easy, reasonably priced and even more, capable of coping with the appetite of a working man or a student.

With our advice the entire family will be able to eat from the same table.

Difficult, you say?!

Certainly, but possible and we will prove it to you.

CHAPTER VI

«FOR» OR «AGAINST» FORBIDDEN FOODS

During these past years we have observed a great many ACCUSATIONS AGAINST THOSE FAMOUS CARBO-HYDRATES IN SEVERAL STUDIES MADE ON OBE-SITY. At first it was sugars, too much salt, or animal fat. So some nutritive compositions were forbidden and others recommended.

With the help of diagrams and complex calculations, a very scientific method has been used to calculate the calories needed to maintain both the body and weight of different sizes and ages.

Everybody has been granted a daily ration of calories, of food, which you are NOT TO EXCEED! IF YOU DON'T want to stay fat or become obese in a short time.

All this is true, and there is no doubt about the credibility of the specialists who worked out these systems and diets.

But in general all this is very difficult to keep up with for a long period if you have a normal family life. Those who have already tried following a strict diet, while sitting down at the table with the others, will know what I mean.

What about the housewife, will she have enough courage, after having cooked for her family, not to taste those delicious, but forbidden, meals?

And for those who resist a little while longer, what is there to say if we consider that unappetizing table, this cooking without imagination, grudged, and without taste?

Ah; the grilled steaks and French beans without butter, cooked whiting without mayonnaise, hard boiled eggs with grated carrots without its vinegar dressing; baked chicken without that crusty skin, without sauce and with a dressing of poached endives!

If this can be tolerated for some time, there comes a moment where these dull meals produce a nasty moral effect.

It may result in a feeling of frustration, or a disliking of food, or jealousy against the lucky ones who can eat whatever they want.

All this is psychological and can even result in the reverse of what we tried to achieve.

The obsession of a diet can provoke optical illusions and, like all emotions, it may impose a strong influence upon the inner being.

So it will disturb, in such a complicated way (that we won't try to explain to your now) what is known as the nutritive centers, whose task it is to regularise our appetite.

This appetite, restrained, ignored, for several weeks, can then become extremely demanding, of the utmost importance, even anarchic.

Then one day, everything breaks down, and we are back to our previous way of nourishment of several years or months ago, together with that sore feeling of having ruined something, of having wasted our time.

We want you to avoid this and so we offer you a simple program. Everybody can do it and it can be kept going for the rest of our life.

CHAPTER VII

LIPIDES (FATS)
CHOOSE THEM WELL,
DON'T EXCLUDE THEM!

Twenty years ago there was a book published in France. It was the translation of a study made by the Hungarian Doctor HERMAN TALLER who had obtained his medical degrees in Italy and afterwards practised in the U.S.A.

This work, although rather revolutionary, didn't create much of an interest at the time. Nevertheless all those who have read it and tried out its, well tested theories, obtained some satisfaction.

In short, the author recommended that a nourishment very heavy in vegetable fats and proteins but poor in carbohydrates, could eventually cause an important reduction of the accumulated fat in tissues.

According to him, some kinds of fats stimulate the organism, not only to burn them up, but even to dispose of the surplus of fat already deposited and spread over the entire body.

It was tempting, but there was a certain danger involved; the overload of the liver, caused by a wrong choice of fatty food, or, by a too sudden change of alimentary customs. If you eat only a little butter or fats, you are not, from one day to another, to triple your ration of fat products, even if they are of vegetable origin. So, even if this theory remains interesting, it can only be of minor importance, and only in order to explain the presence of a certain quantity of these products, in our recommended amounts. Even this might surprise or confuse you.

In fact, in this book you won't find specific chapter dealing with so called « DIET-PRODUCTS », such as « wheat-germs, yeast, soyaflour, several exotic fruits, american cheeses, rare exotic spices etc. »; All this you can buy, if you want to, in specialised shops, but let us tell you right away, that, as a matter of fact, all those products are only replacing the ones which are grown in our country and which have almost the same qualities and nourishing values.

What we suggest to you is to use alimentary products of « our own », even regional ones, which are easy to find, taste nice and are pleasing to the eye, because they are related to all kinds of family and social customs.

Yes, give the Choucroute to the Alsacians, the creme to the Normans, the fish to the Bretons, preserved fruit to the Gascons, garlic and olives to the inhabitants of Provence.

And all this together, to the French, who are a mixture of all these regions, and who will certainly find their own needs and roots.

CHAPTER VIII

THE MAJOR KEY: LIVING HAPPILY

There can't be any question of you losing weight and at the same time losing your happiness for living, this would be the wrong way to do it.

If it should happen that you decide to diminish or avoid some bad habits, you must be able to do so « with joy ». Never say to yourself Although I love pork chops with cream sauce, unfortunately, I must deny it to myself. Poor me! Why « Poor You »? Why « Deny »? You'd better say: han turkey fillets, stuffed with spinach, steamed in a little butter and lemon, delicious! I would eat it with pleasure. (You 'll find the recipe further on).

Don't be sad over one cocktail less or an orange juice you bought at the store and which you'd better avoid.

They can easily be replaced by a glass of good wine or by an orange you pressed yourself. It's very nice too.

In fact, stop thinking about the things you won't eat anymore (or very little) because they won't be worth mentioning. But think of ALL the things you can eat. And the amount of products still at your entire disposal is CONSIDERABLE, you'd better believe it.

Enough of the « TREAT YOU AND YOUR ENTIRE FAMILY » as it is said in commercials with one difference though, you won't be guided by an advertisement for cheese, drinks or frozen meals, but it will be YOU who decides and does the shopping so as to meet your daily alimentary program.

These purchases will contain all the needs for the well-being of the entire body, and, as everybody knows, it means:
— Vegetable and animal proteins.
— Carbo-hydrates in a form of sugar and starches.
— Fats, preferably vegetable (polyunsaturated margarine, sunflower and olive oil).
— Fruits and vegetables to be eaten raw or slightly cooked. In this way your meals will contain a sufficient amount of vitamins; as they are found in almost all fresh foods.

We point out to you that, should you be interested, you can find lists of vitamins in every drugstore or health food shop.

So, up till now, NOTHING has been changed in your feeding habits.

You leave for the market, and you have the intention to give your family healthy and satisfactory nourishment, while, at the same time, little by little, you will eliminate some of that extra fat of yours, without exaggerated restrictions.

What will you buy now?

CHAPTER IX

YOUR SHOPPING

I – IT'S A PLEASURE

First of all be in a good moood when you go shopping. Just like all the other different chores there are to do around the house, this also is a very important and interesting moment, as in fact you're buying LIFE AND HEALTH for your family.

And like everything important, you are to think about it in advance and, if possible, draw up a list of all the things you need.

It will be a restricted list because, while making it up, you will deliberately omit industrial products, which might tempt you, Pre-cooked meals, which have only to be heated (Sandwich - meats - cakes etc.). And, if you are determined enough, you will not mention all those things you're so fond of or those things your husband can't get enough of (it it is he who has to slim).

If those products Don't Figure On Your List, you won't think of buving them.

Take the precaution to go shopping in the early morning. You know why? Because, if you just had an elaborate breakfast, you won't be hungry and so not be tempted by tarts or pork-butcher's meat, whereas if you leave about II a.m. it will become difficult, as breakfast is already long forgotten and your stomach demands more.

This will make you succumb to every folly, starting from rolls up to some real cream paté. Temptations that are better to be avoided.

As we told you at the beginning of this chapter.

« Do your shopping in a good mood ».

It is important!!

Because, first of all, happiness is dynamic. It makes you feel light, walk supple, stand up straight. It wakes your dynamics, and ALERT DYNAMICS MAKES FAT MELT! So many women do their shopping without joy, already nervous, tired. They wander around shops, not knowing what to buy, or else, rushed by time, grab anything at all, especially those things easy to prepare, if it does't turn out to be the eternal pre-wrapped ham slices or frozen meals.

Remember well, that, what you are doing is very *important,* but it certainly isn't forbiddent to combine the agreeable with the useful.

The agreeable is the smell of fruit, fresh herbs, colors of cans and packages and, why not, even the penetrating scent of cheese.

No, shopping isn't tiresome at all, certainly not if you have the chance of having a market place in the open, with all its joyful noises.

Who wouldn't enjoy it?

Isn't there a poem, we learned a long time ago at school, that said:

> « By the rising of the sun,
>   on the small square
> The market laughs happily, noisy
>   colourful and fair ».

56

II – SUPPLIES AND PRIORITIES

Maybe you do your shopping only two or three times a week? The importance and quality of our modern refrigerators allow us to preserve meat and dairy products for about three days. Nevertheless, if possible, always try to eat «fresh» vegetables and fruit. They already came a long way, from originally being picked, before being sold, so it is better not to delay any further their consumption.

So, on the same day as your shopping, your menu should include fragile fruits: strawberrys, cherries, peaches, grapes, ripe bananas. More solid fruits such as: apples, oranges, pears, are to be eaten the second or third day.

The same goes for vegetables.

The first day is the one you serve baby peas, tomatoes, asparagus; French beans, spinach, salads or mushrooms.

Until the second day you can keep: endives, cabbages, cucumber, aubergines. The third day is reserved for carrots and potatoes.

You will proceed the same way for cheeses: first white cheese (or whipped cheese) - yoghurts - Petit Suisses, and fermented cheese (roquefort - blue cheeses - camembert-brie).

Then come cheeses of a more solid composition: gruyere - gouda - port salut - cantal goat cheese.

As for meat, we usualy put it in the ice box (3 stars), if we don't have a freezer. There it can be kept for quite some time. The thing to do, is first to remove the fat as it proves to be dificult to preserve in cold surroundings.

If you have neither a freezer nor a 3 star ice box, you must know that your ordinary fridge will only keep your meat edible for about three days. In this case you must also use priorities: on the first day eat veal and chicken, keep beef and mutton for the next day.

Concerning non-frozen fish, it has to be eaten: THE SAME DAY.

Nourishment is never complete if it doesn't include eggs. So you will buy some while shopping.

You know that whether you look at the package date or trust your shop-keeper, you'll never have the so called « FRESH LAID EGGS ».

But as it is protected by its delicate but solid shell, the egg will keep longer than any other food.

Nevertheless, we advise you to keep them no longer than one week. That's why it is better to buy only the quantity that is required to prepare your meal: scrambled eggs, fried eggs or cakes.

The egg that was « TOO MUCH » - or forgotten in the fridge and then used the day we were short of fresh ones, can cause slight food poisoning.

So, no supply of eggs, only the necessary amount.

In short, you must try to make a shopping-list providing meals for three consecutive days. This list has to be drawn up carefully bearing in mind all the advice we gave you.

This will guarantee you, as far as possible, the freshnes of food products you are to eat together with your family.

III – FRESH FOOD PRODUCTS

THE CHOICE of food products is the starting point of the change you are about to tackle.

We will not use words such as: « SUPPRESSION » that can be sad and traumatising but rather talk about « SUBSTITUTION » that will be clearly more positive. So, don't say: « I'd rather buy a goose, but it's too fattening; I'm not supposed to eat it but say: « roast chicken, that's very good and what's more the children love it »!

As we told you in chapter VIII you can make your choice from a very elaborate and almost endless list of alimentary products: such as:

Vegetables:

You can have them all. The only thing to do is to eat them fresh and property prepared (we will come back to this later on). Just go easy on the potatoes, but everybody knows that!

Fruits

Tangerines, grape-fruits, pine-apples, oranges, currants, strawberries, raspberries. Don't weigh them, but eat them every day if you like (further on we will tell you when and how to eat them).

In a more moderate way, except for your children, you can eat: apricots, peaches, nectarines, apples, black grapes, pears and plums.

With such a large choice you are bound to forget the existence of bananas, and mangoes. But in fact, you are not so fond of them, are you?

59

Meat

Here also you have a large variety. What, will you tell us, don't you talk about excluding pork and mutton? NO!! All these different kinds of meat can figure on your menu once a day, but, where you are concerned, under certain conditions. Those conditions will be explained to you during the next chapter.

Poultry and eggs

No exceptions either, but, here also, prepared in a certain way.

Fish

You can eat them all, as they are very healthy for your whole family. Yes, even herring and sardines.

Dairy products

Although they are of great necessity for the nutrition of young ones, they are less important to adults.

Nevertheless you can eat them when they are on the table. You won't be able to avoid this, if you are one of those « cheese minded » families. But there again you will be told later on what to do exactly.

What you are to avoid is: sweetened yoghourt, ice-creams, or full-cream milk between meals, or during meals you have alone.

IV – OTHER INGREDIENTS

Adding the six different kinds of ingredients we just talked about, we noticed that there are many others which will add or mix well with your daily menu. They are needed for cooking, flavouring or to be served with your main dish. Further on we will give you some reasons to be cautions.

Sugar and honey

You need only a little, like everybody else, but then you find it in fresh fruit and bread. So, your sugar lumps will be counted and honey served drop-wise. But you will see, it's not difficult to do.

Bread and starchy food

Generally every kind of bread has the same nutritious value. As well as rusks. Sometimes they even show traces of excessive fat. SO BUY THE BREAD YOU LIKE, but, EAT JUST ONE SLICE AT MEAL TIMES.

Always, take small bites, chew well, so it is mixed up thoroughly with the food it is served with.

And noodles?

They may not exceed 5% of your nourishment. But if you must cook them your family? How will you manage? We will explain to you later on.

Pastries

They are not to be banished from your kitchen, although you will have to learn to reserve them for your children.

It is understood that we talk about home-made pastry or made by a conscientious pastry-cook.

As for you, eat them little as possible.

Jam

This is for the children. As well as milk chocolate or rich chocolates. You'd do better to eat marmelade and lightly sweetened apple compote and pears, and a piece of pure chocolate.

Fats

They are: butter, sunflower margerine, sunflower oil, (as it is dear to the Southerners) Olive oil can be used as salad dressing.

Drinks

You can drink wine, beer, and water. But try to avoid sweet gassy drinks, mild cocktails; sparkling water, sweet cider. In fact all that is commercially prepared.

Spices

Here we have a wide choice, and can use all natural spices, which perfume and appetize your meals. In ancient times they had to be fetched from miles away, in spite of danger, and their price was high.

First of all there are HERBS: thyme, chives, parsley, garlic, tarragon, chervil etc.

Then comes spices in grains or in powder: pepper, juniper-berry, cinnamon etc. Use them correctly.

So, we have almost completed our shopping.

You can see that only a few things have to be changed. Isn't this encouraging?

CHAPTER X

WHAT TO EAT? WHERE? WHEN? HOW?

1 – WHAT TO EAT?

As we have said previously, you can use everyday products except: Animal Fats, bacon, lard (anyway they are not appreciated in France), Smoked Fish, Smoked Meat, Jam, Bananas, Sweet Gassy Drinks, Pre-Cooked Meals, or Sauces, which are not really indispensable.

So you can feed your family without depriving anybody of anything at all. Anyway, it's only to be benefit of your entire family if you decide to cut down drastically on all those ingredients we mentioned before.

Exceptions are to be made for « real » jam where children are concerned. On one condition: they shouldn't become chubby, this has to be watched closely. You will notice that you are left with quite a choice of allowed food products, and that the shopping we did together previously, contains no restriction whatsoever where the choice of products is concerned.

But now we have to know how to prepare correctly, and in optimal condition, this food we bought.

2 – WHERE TO EAT?

This question may make you smile, but it has its importance. Eating, just like sleeping or practising sports, isn't done just anywhere.

AT HOME, it may be in the kitchen, dining room or on the balcony, whether you are on your own or with family, set your table as appealingly as possible. Meals are a good time for you to relax, to sit down in front of a colorful dish, a sparkling glass, a clean table-cloth, it's already the beginning of a pleasant chapter of your daily life.

With the lack of a table-cloth, a plastified one will do just as well. Choose it in pink or green as those two colors give you an appetite.

« Give an appetite? »!! « But surely », you will say, « This is not what I need! »

Ah! But you do really! Promoting an appetite starts the saliva going, which is required for good digestion.

We will see later on that a good digestion slows down formation of alimentary wastes and extra fat.

So, it is good to be *hungry* while sitting down at the table.

For those of you, WHO EAT out; canteen, cafeteria, restaurant, a special chapter for you alone, will follow. But from now on you must know that, during Summertime, you will find it much more pleasant to eat your own home-made salad on a bench in the square or by a river bank watching birds.

But there again it's your choice. If you love the atmosphere in your cafeteria, don't change your habits, at least not when it concerns the locale.

Breakfast

Let us reveal a *secret,* you are not to have your breakfast just anywhere, on the corner of the table, or standing in front of your sink. Numerous women do so, in order to gain time, after having served their husband and children, or out of laziness or just to nibble « a little something » with their coffee.

This is a GREAT MISTAKE. *This is* what we encourage you to do, starting from tomorrow morning:

Waking up, have a WARM, and sweet drink (non fat chocolate milk or chicory and milk), and GO BACK TO BED!! FOR ANOTHER TEN MINUTES!!! RELAX...

Proceeding this way start up the eliminatory mechanism of your bowels. Their peristaltic motion can even force you to go to the toilet. Once this formality is taken care of, get dressed, then prepare a real breakfast for your husband and children if they have to leave the house before you. If you work too and have to leave early, or if for one reason or another you can't do otherwise, have breakfast with them, but SIT DOWN at the table and take it easy. Why should they and not you?

Make the children remove their own dirty dishes and put them into the sink. It's the least they can do!!

It would be better though to have your breakfast, AFTER THEY'VE GONE, because then you can eat as you want to, much more relaxed.

Further on, you'll find the right way to prepare this breakfast. A breakfast is so important, and yet so much neglected these days.

3 – WHEN TO EAT???

The Hours of Our Meals

Meals should be served when we are hungry. That's how, at the beginning, men were conditioned. But, little by little, human digestive functions were altered radically by social or family rules, working hours, transportation schedules and spare time.

So, man learned to feed himself at regular times, whether he's hungry or not, his stomach empty or still digesting his previous meal.

These hours are those which match best one's occupations, working hours at the office or factory; children's school-work and even. T.V. programs!!!

So, we have learned to eat regularly 3 or 4 times a day, and our organism, marvellously supple and adjustable, accepts this rhythm and forces itself to receive, digest, assimilate and eliminate at well determined times. All this is true for almost any civilised family.

It's up to the housewife to find « THE GENTLE WAY » to have her family eat together at a time that suits everyone and that matches cooking hours. In order to avoid friction, and nervous tension, have BREAKFAST at that precise hour which enables everybody to enjoy it, nobody will have to rush into the streets still chewing.

AT NOON, some eat out. For those who eat at home, have the meal ready on time, so it will be possible to have about 1/4 hour left over to relax.

This dinner should be WITHOUT FUSS and EASY TO PREPARE.

TEA, this small, but traditional, meal is excellent for children, but IF IT IS WELL CHOSEN, it can also be good for an adult, who is systematically reducing his main meals.

So we can include « TEA » into your anti-fat program.

From a psychological point of view it's SUPPER that constitutes the most pleasant moment of the day (where it concerns served meals) for the entire family.

There also, once the time is set to an hour convenient for everybody, not omitting the cook, we must try to cling to it.

So, if we decide to have supper at 8p.m., let us have it at 8p.m., and no later. Everybody has to have at least 1 hour of relaxation before going to bed.

We have mentioned the *readiness* of the cook. If she stays at home, it's easy for her to have meals ready on time.

But those who go out to work, must have at least 1 hour at their disposal, in order to get the main meal ready. To those people we will suggest, later on, very special meals (for the evenings).

She also must be able to sit down and enjoy this family meal, without being nervous or in a hurry.

4 – HOW TO EAT

If we insist upon having a CALM atmosphere during family meals, it's because we know how hard THIS is to achieve!!!

Everybody's nerves have been through a great deal after a day's work, travelling here and there by bus or on the subway, surrounded by noise and agitation.

This exhaustion shows mostly, especially with children, by overexcitement; parents usually react by being somewhat exasperated!!!

The atmosphere at home can be very tense some nights!!!

A meal, eaten in such an atmosphere, will most likely be tiring and boring. In order to talk, argue or even quarrel, we swallow mouthfuls without chewing, swallowing as much air as food, breathe wrongly, the plexus remains tense. All this is followed by difficult digestion, aerophagia, interrupted sleep, wrong co-ordination.

The chemical process of digestion is difficult. The food, not disintegrated enough, is difficult to digest. The liver has a hard time, fulfulling its important functions. The organism can't master all this anymore, and the surplus of unused fat will be integrated in the tissues.

It would be nice if you could have your meals in a PEACEFUL atmosphere while THINKING ABOUT WHAT YOU'RE DOING.

In monasteries where meals are very sober, containing only: bread, cooked vegetables, and a small portion of meat, the monks seem to be very strong and healthy. They have very important physical and intellectual duties to fulfil (working-cleaning-studies-walks...) and yet you will never find them to be tired, nervous or depressed.

There are 2 reasons for this: their spiritual life which grants them an unusual moral force and a very rational way of nourishment that guarantees a perfect absorption of the food by the entire body.

The meal is taken IN SILENCE, each bite is THOROUGHLY CHEWED, the food is eaten WITH RESPECT.

This way all nutritious substances are well impregnated by saliva and other digestive juices which give a perfect digestion.

NOTHING IS LOST, the food takes up its role of providing the organism with « FUEL » by producing a maximum of energy and leaving only a minimum of waste.

AT ANY TIME, let us keep this example in mind.

Doctor P. Carter, who, some 10 years ago, tried to teach the French to eat more conscientiously, advised them to CHEW 15 UP TO 20 TIMES EACH BITE. This way, a simple piece of bread could TASTE differently 5 or 6 times while chewing it.

There is no need to be so extreme, but we must know that by CHEWING MORE, WE EAT LESS, and still are satisfied.

All taste and aroma is developed IN THE MOUTH. So, why deny yourself this pleasure by swallowing in a hurry?

CHAPTER XI

EAT: HOW MUCH?

When the only thing that matters is to lose weight progressively, but what is more, in a PERMANENT way, while keeping up a normal active life, we certainly can't start weighing scrupulously steaks, cheese, or potatoes.

Nevertheless, there's no harm done, if you are able to evaluate the nutritous value of a food product, by the mere sight of it.

Of course, there are people who want to lose weight VERY QUICKLY, even if it is only to start off their « losing weight » programme well. Some feel the need to strengthen their intentions of slimming, by the fact that it is possible. Therefore they need to SEE, and see RIGHT AWAY, the scale needle bend in the right direction. They might be deceived when we talk about a progressive, but continuous, way of losing weight. It's for those people, and for them only, that we will indicate, at the end of this book, menus of a very restricted quantity, which have to observed for a short while (5 days at the most) under certain conditions.

As for us, we prefer a less spectacular start, but a more progressive and secure way for regaining our ideal shape. This we intend to do by what is called « THE PLATE SYSTEM ».

75

THE PLATE SYSTEM

Let us give you a example: When you serve: veal fricassee, creole rice, and steamed carrots, you should be able to estimate in advance, by a simple look, the quantity of meat, how many spoonfuls of rice and carrots, it takes to feed yourself, WITHOUT YOUR PUTTING ON WEIGHT. As for sauce, containing flour and egg yolks, leave it, as much as possible, to the others.

The average piece of meat weighs about 1½ oz. and contains approximately 1/3 oz. of proteins. You're allowed 2 pieces of meat only.

Rice is rich in carbohydrates. Together with the meat it's better to go easy on it, about 3 spoonfuls). Instead serve yourself some more carrots. (The equivalent of 2 whole carrots).

So from this delicious meal, that pleases your entire family, you can have up to the amount of a small cheese plate. If, at the same time, a salad of green vegetables is being served, you can help yourself up to the amount of a small ladle.

You will also eat 1 slice of bread - 1 piece of cheese (1¼" x 1").

Let's recapitulate: if you ESTIMATE in advance what you are to eat in order to satisfy your appetite; keep your body healthy, without putting on weight, whilst at the same time diminish your « excess-weight », you will find that it takes not much but the CONTENTS OF A PLATE.

Yes, salad, meat, vegetables or pastas, bread and cheese; it must all BE KEEPT ON ONE PLATE!!

Try to measure it several times in a row, by putting YOUR ENTIRE MEAL on a normal plate.

Remove, without hesitation, all the superfluous, and don't cheat by piling things up!! DON'T use an extra large plate, but take the usual one (10" diameter).

When you have put next to each other 6 tomato slices or 3 spoonfuls of red cabbage salad, 1/2 hard boiled egg, 1 small escalope, 1 spoonful of French beans, 2 small roasted potatoes, 1 piece of cheese, Only THEN will you have an example of what should satisfy your appetite. Little by little, you will get used to these quantities and you will notice that these quantities are sufficient, as in fact, you can have a little of everything.

What is more, the idea will settle in your subconcious and you will have NO URGE whatsoever to have more. Everything that might be served extra to you, will seem to be SUPERFLUOUS.

« What about dessert », you will ask. Is it not included in this kind of military ration?

NO, dessert, usually consists of fancy cakes (if they are served right after your main meal, you are to leave them to the others) in fact you shouldn't have any at all for now; or fruit (fruit should be eaten at least 1½ hours after meals).

This PLATE RATION SYSTEM is very simple and efficient. It will become automatic very soon and it's far from being as boring as weighing every little thing or making complex calculations of calories. Everybody can do it and the system can be used for A LIFE TIME, for every possible occasion: family meals, canteens, dinner parties. It's the EYE that weighs, chooses, it evaluates the necessary quantity of each article of food, as efficiently as it evaluates distances when driving a car. Most importantly this system is very discreet. You can have your « anti-fat » diet without anybody noticing it, because you can still eat almost everything.

CHAPTER XII

CHEWING

Before getting to the more practical part of this book, we must, once more, insist upon this very important item: MASTICATION.

Together with the idea of VISUALISING your PLATE MEAL, it is one of the most fundamental principles of keeping your exact weight.

In fact, if you think twice, you will notice that: EVERYTHING concerning your digestion, once your food passed the gullet, is out of control.

The process of food, the mixing of the entire food mass, the work done by gastric juices, the slow brewing in the small intestine, the complicated chemical process that results in producing the energy to keep your entire body healthy, followed by waste excretion of this chemical process; all this is done without you being aware of it, you have no choice in the matter.

But, what are we trying to do here? Well, to have a real effect on what we CAN control. Shopping, cooking, proportioning food on a plate, time and atmosphere during meals, absorption of food. Our ACTIVE PART ends here. So it's UP TO US to be as efficient as possible.

We won't tell you, as Doctor Carton did, to chew each bite 20 times and this from tomorrow on (although you can do it if you really want to) but we will tell you to observe yourself while you eat. Most people from our country, which has a large variety of food products, take it all for granted and eat indifferently. After having chosen their menu, looked at their meal furtively (maybe, if we are lucky, smelled the pleasant aroma of a « spécialité culinaire ») they begin swallowing their food. Their thoughts are miles away. Sometimes they even talk or read while eating. So, in 3 mouthfuls, or a quick swallow, everything is eaten.

Is this your way of eating? Maybe. If this is so, you must learn, from now on, to chew longer each time, to turn your food round and round in your mouth so it mixes up well with saliva to form a pulp. Once your food is like this you can swallow it.

Of course, it will take you more than one day to do so. Even so, should you try to double or even triple your mastications at once, your jaws would most certainly start to hurt, not being used to so much gymnastics.

So, take it easy at first. If you are already in the habit of chewing your food 3 times, try to do it now once or twice more. You will notice that bread or meat takes about at least 10 to 12 mastications in order to be reduced into pulp.

But once you have started to « think » about your mastication, you will be at first surprised by its importance, then convinced rapidly, about its almost miraculous influence on your digestion.

But that's not all, and once again we draw your attention to 2 secondary, but remarkable, results, this long and thorough mastication will have:
1) It will make you eat slowly, and so it will take you longer to finish your meal. You won't feel the need to serve yourself twice.
2) You will quickly have a sensation of satisfaction and well-being. You will have the impression of really having

eaten « very well » and « more than sufficient ». You
will have had the benefit af each mouthful, of each flavor,
You will, physically and psychologically be pleased by
your meal.

In short, once more we advise: CHEW BETTER,
YOU'LL EAT LESS and DIGEST PERFECTLY.

BASIC PRINCIPLES

The time has come to recapitulate all we have learned
during previous chapters. What are those basic ideas we have
to remember well, in order to stop or reduce an embarras-
sing obesity, without suffering, being tired, incurring costs
and discouragements?

1) Let's write down all the pro's and contra's and decide
   whether or not we must slim.

2) Fix our IDEAL WEIGHT and draw up a REAL
   IMAGE of how we want to be (or be again). According
   to this we will know many pounds will have to disappear.

3) Write down our menus and shopping lists in accordance
   to the needs of our family and leave out all animal fat,
   industrial sugars, sweetened gassy drinks, precooked
   meals.

4) Let's try to have our meals at regular times, in a calm,
   restful and most importantly a friendly atmosphere.

5) We must make a habit of chewing our food more, so we
   have a maximum of energy and a minimum of waste.

6) Reduce the quantity of food, eaten during 2 principal
   meals, to the contents of 1 PLATE... and without chea-
   ting.

Amongst those principles, there are 3 you are never to forget, as they should become your best qualities, here they are:

— calmess, good mood during meals
— long and careful mastication
— evaluating, by the PLATE SYSTEM, the necessary, and sufficient food quantity.

We don't think you'll have any difficulty assimilating the above information as in fact all this is mere WISDOM and GOOD SENSE.

From now on you must be perfectly relaxed, determined, « in a gentle way », to deal with your problem of overweight.

Now, we will study together, the more practical side, the COOKING to be exact, it will help you to shape up again this marvellous machine known as your body.

CHAPTER XIII

COOKING

We saw how to plan menus for 3 consecutive days.

Once the food-stuffs are duly stocked in a chronological way, according to their utilisation (ref. Chapter IX first part) we now have to use them and learn how to prepare them in a correct way.

1) Meat

— Where you are concerned, you are to have but a small portion each day ($\pm$ 3 oz./5 oz.).

— You should have it lightly cooked, even veal, that may stay slightly pink.

— Remove most of the fat and add no butter into the frying-pan when you BEGIN frying. The fat of the meat itself should be sufficient. If not, or in order to baste it, add 1 or 2 spoonfuls of lukewarm water.

— No sauces to go with your meat (certainly not if they contain: wine, alcohol, or cream). The human liver isn't fond of it (later on we will give you details about proper sauces).

2) Fish

— There also, avoid too sophisticated sauces. Spices, herbs, a slice of lemon will do.

— For cooking in the oven, don't use any fat, but put the fish on a bed of tomatoes, which will provide juices. Half way through cooking sprinkle it with ½ glass of lemon juice (some water added).

— In order to fry fish, (or fish fillets) you must dry and coat them well in flour. Put I spoonful of sunflour oil in a frying-pan, once the fish is well browned remove all remaining oil and finish the cooking.

3) Poultry

— Chicken-Turkey, contain enough proteins and fats to ensure a nourishing meal. You can prepare them either in the oven or in a Tefal pan, without any addition of fat. (as you know, poultry fat melts and settles to the bottom of the pan).

— Remove the fat — juices and replace them by water to make your sauce. If you don't want to dispose of all the fat, you can keep a small part of it ($\pm$ 1/3) in the fridge to use later on.

— After having poured water on your poultry, leave it to finish baking on a moderate heat. When it's done, glaze by adding lemon juice.

4) Eggs

— From time to time you can eat ½ a boiled egg as a dressing for any uncooked food. But in general you should reserve fried eggs or omelets for meals without meat or fish.

— FRIED EGGS (1 for you, 2 for the others) are prepared in a Tefal pan, which is SLIGHTLY OILED (1 teaspoon of sunflower oil for 6 eggs) or in a slightly WET pan (if you do so, have your eggs baked over a small fire and COVER THEM UP: they will fry better).

— The omelet can be cooked in exactly the same way. In order to make it more digestable REPLACE 1 in 4 eggs by 2 spoonfuls of whipped cheese (0% fat). BEFORE pouring everything in a pan: stir up the eggs and cheese, add the chosen ingredients (tomato sauce, onions, ham, cheese or spinach). This is very IMPORTANT: NEVER pour beaten eggs on an ingredient already baking in a pan.

— Delicious egg recipes will be given to you later.

5) Vegetables

You will eat them RAW or SLIGHTLY COOKED

— RAW: wash them carefully, scrub them, slice into thin strips, and eat them for a salad. If you serve your vegetables thinly sliced, you will have a double advantage: firstly better mastication and secondly the volume will SEEM TO BE GREATER. This way you will eat less of them. You can eat raw: carrots, cucumbers, radishes, chicory, tomatoes, peppers, cabbage, celery, Paris mushrooms, cauliflower, and of course all green salads.

— STEAMED: Don't think you'll have to buy expensive utensils in order to steam your vegetables. Should you have them, good for you. Otherwise, you can steam your vegetables in slightly salted boiling water for about 10 to 15 minutes.

This way you can have: baby peas, French beans, diced carrots, asparagus, courgettes, onions, cabbage, leak, sliced chicory, cauliflower, all these vegetables can be served with several dressings.

Here also, this way of preparing vegetables, diced or sliced, is at the same time economic (they are tender much sooner) and dietetic (increased taste and less quantity).

We can tell you that this is one of the special (and most attractive) characteristics of the « nouvelle cuisine » which is practised by all our « Great Chefs ».

— POTATOES: Are treated separately. We will give you some special recipes later concerning their cooking as a sole vegetable or to be eaten with other vegetables.

6) Starches

Pastas, rice, wheat or maize flour must be in your family meal. What would become of us without them? But we must state, once and for all, that where you are concerned, they may represent only 20% of your total alimentation.

But how are we to calculate what this represents in quantity and is weight? This is the time to memorise your plateration: a small place is reserved for:

bread: 1 small slice
potatoes: 3 small ones
pastas, semolina or rice: 3 spoonfuls.

— HOW TO COOK THEM

Don't use salted water, but water FLAVOURED with 1 clove, a pinch of thyme or celerysalt.

Once the water is boiling let them simmer for about ¼ hour - drain the water and spice.

For cooking noodles, you can use the water you used to steam your vegetables. They will taste better and regain some of the mineral salts dissolved in the water while cooking.

90

— If those starches are to be served with meat (which is a common in our country) always remember to serve greens with it. You will take 2 spoonfuls of greens for I spoonful of starches.

7) Potatoes

As we have said previously, they can figure in our menus, but only when they are to be served with other vegetables; or as a « single dish ».

The only BIG sacrifice you have to make, is never to eat any French fried potatoes (chips) again. You can still eat them with skins, cooked or steamed in the oven with milk. In order to eat less of them, serve them with carrots, French beans or cabbage.

As you can see, the use and preparation of starches, is the part that demands most of our attention. You dont have to scrap them totally from your menu, except during the days you've decided to follow a light diet.

If possible you should eat them alone or served with greens.

AVOID AS MUCH AS POSSIBLE TO EAT THEM WITH MEAT OR FISH. If you can't do otherwise only have a little, and eat more green vegetables served with them.

CHAPTER XIV

SOME MORE DETAILS

1) Hot meals? Cold meals?

It is best to eat soups and starches fairly warm, meat and vegetables tepid (luke warm), tea and coffee warm and without sugar, wine, water, beer and fruit juices should be at room temperature.

We have already told you that sweets and ice-cream are forbidden to you, so we won't mention them here.

Think about your stomach, it doesn't like receiving hot or icy liquids as this interferes with its work: remember this!

2) Left – Overs

In books dealing with « economic housekeeping » it is always recommended to avoid waste. So we invented « THE ART OF PREPARING LEFTOVERS » in which our mothers and grand-mothers were real experts. Who doesn't remember the old slices of bread turned into a delicious pudding or French fried? Leftover broth, or beef and carrots, turned into a stew, or a beef casserole, and meatballs made of dried out leftovers of roast meat?

Even today these old family recipes come in handy, as they can still be improved and used frequently.

BUT BE CAREFUL: leftovers of cold meats or stews can't be kept much longer than 24 hours in the fridge. So these meals prepared from leftovers should be prepared the very next day.

3) Pastries

Our advice to you was, to eat them as little as possible, as they are extremely nutritious and contain all the necessary ingredients of a normal meal.

Did you know that a cake is nothing more than a concentration of starches sugars and fat? Sometimes cakes even contain dried fruits or nuts!, so, you must know that 2 slices of cake and 1 glass of milk have the same nutritious equivalent as an ENTIRE MEAL! So, if you had this kind of tea at about 4.30 p.m., your supper has to be less important than usual, in order to keep your food balance.

4) Fruit

All dieticians agree on saying that fruit doesn't go very well with meat, as it prevents the digestion of carbo-hydrates. So, in order to avoid this, we suggest that you should have your fruit at a time IN BETWEEN MEALS and EATEN ALONE. This means: mornings: ± 10 a.m., afternoons: ± 4 p.m., evenings: ± 10.30 p.m. Your fruit will seem much more fresh and tasty.

5) Raw foods

Bite size raw foods and green salad, are to be served at the beginning of a meal, eat it together with HALF a slice of bread, and CHEW IT WELL in order to reduce each mouthful into a pulp.

6) Healthy Diet

At the beginning of this book we have told you how dangerous a continuous fast, without supervision, can be.

But if you are feeling somewhat oppressive or uneasy (after a social dinner or after holidays) treat yourself to a LIGHT MEAL DAY:

— vegetable broth
— poached egg
— soft cheese
— stewed fruit

and drink only lemon-flavored water. The next day you will feel much better. Except if you are ill, you are NEVER TO STAY A WHOLE DAY WITHOUT FOOD.

CHAPTER XV

SOME MENU IDEAS

In order to help you, we have written down some menus to be used during your first weeks, they have a large choice of meat and vegetables that you can alter and improve as you like. It is understood that changes must occur according to seasons and choice.

First you will find some ideas for a healthy breakfast with very little sweet food products, but instead, the presence of food such as meat or cheese. In fact, jam or honey, containing sugar, is quickly digested, and this will give you a very unpleasant feeling of hunger at about 11 a.m.

Next we will give you a series of menus containing meat or fish WITHOUT STARCHES but WITH GREEN VEGETABLES.

Next a series of menus WITH VEGETABLES and STARCHES but WITHOUT MEAT.

For dinner or supper you'll choose a meal according to your preference, needs and time schedules.

It all depends on family customs; the number of meals taken together, the quality and quantity of meals eaten out by each of them.

If you had a light dinner out, you can still have a more consistant supper containing MEAT or FISH. But, if your dinner out was heavier, choose a menu without meat but with STARCHES.

101

As we have already told you, meat should preferably be served with green vegetables without starches. But as we know this could cause problems for a family; we can only advise you once more, don't eat them YOURSELF. If you have noodles or potatoes, serve them alone or with vegetables.

BREAKFAST

Of course you will remember to put only ½ *lump of sugar* in the drink you have chosen for breakfast, as you had already a warm sweetened drink ½ hour before, in order to ease the intestinal functions.

Some examples for breakfast (containing little fat)
milk with chicory
2 rusks with gluten
low-fat butter or sunflower margarine

———

black coffee
ripened cheese (emmenthal, comté, mimolette)
1 slice of bread

———

tea with a little fresh milk
1 toasted slice of bread
compote of fresh apples

———

coffee with milk
1 rusk - 1 slice of ham

Non-fat chocolate milk
1 slice of whole-wheat bread
lightly buttered

———

black coffee
1 soft boiled egg - 1 slice of bread

———

fresh fruit juice
1 slice of bread - a small piece of unsweetened chocolate

———

lemon tea
1 slice of toasted bread
1 baked apple without sugar

———

black coffee
1 rusk, 1 slice of Dutch cheese

———

milk
1 slice of gluten bread,
some cooked prunes

———

broth
1 breadroll, 1 small pack cream cheese (petit-suisse)

fruit juice
1 buttered rusk
some honey

———

tea with milk
1 fried egg (without fat)
1 small slice of bread

———

black coffee
compote of pears, 2 rusks

———

coffee with milk
1 rusk with some low-fat butter and roquefort cheese

———

lemon tea
toasted bread or rusk
1 soft boiled egg

———

fruit juice
1 lightly sugared bun

———

As you can see, where breakfast is concerned, you can let your imagination do the work. Surely, even your children will appreciate this change of menu.

EXAMPLES OF MEALS CONTAINING MEAT OR FISH

Mixed green salad
lamb chops
green beans or broad beans
camembert

———

stuffed raw tomatoes
roast or veal with carrots (see recipe)
brie

———

a salad of asparagus or French beans
roasted chicken, tomatoes " provencal "

———

radish, a little butter, sausage (1 ring, for you)
cod cooked with vegetables
(carrots, French beans, cauliflower)
cream cheese

———

salad niçoise
beefburger
small potatoes with some parsley butter

green salad, with bits of toast and minced hard boiled eggs
fried fish fillets
braised chicory
yoghurt

———

chinese salad (see recipe)
rabbit with mustard
potatoes and carrots
gruyère cheese

———

red cabbage - vinaigrette dressing
cheese and ham omelet
Baked courgettes au gratin (see recipe)
soft cheese

———

ham roll (see recipe)
mushroom and potatoe waffles
creamcheese (petit suisse)

———

Provencal salad
roast beef
baked spinach
camembert

———

leek with vinaigrette
fried chicken, tomatoes and mushrooms
brie or camembert

stuffed avocado
escalope with lemon
ratatouille
gruyere

« slim » salad (see recipe)
light sauerkraut
youghurt

---

minced eggs with parsley
grilled liver
steamed aubergines
roquefort cheese

---

chicory salad
steak with mustard
baked cauliflower with potatoes
soft cream cheese

All these examples are only to help you, you are free to change them as much as you like; But always keep in mind the elementary principles we mentioned before.

As to sweets, remember that they are forbidden to you, not to the others!

EXAMPLES OF MEALS WITHOUT MEAT BUT WITH VEGETABLES AND STARCHES

Mushrooms à la Grecque
Gratin Dauphinois
cheese - youghurt

―――

vegetable broth
spaghetti and tomatoes
baked apples

―――

A choice of vegetables with 1 hard boiled egg
soft cheese

―――

Gratin d'aubergines
créole rice
custard

―――

celery with herb sauce
cauliflower - potatoes - bechamel sauce
yoghurt or cheese

―――

green salad
stuffed tomatoes and peppers

potato salad
leek quiche (see recipe)
cheese

———

chicory with sauce
potato croquettes (see recipe)
gruyere cheese

———

mixed vegetable salad
toasted ham and cheese sandwich
compote of apples or pears

———

mixed salad (chicory, gruyere, potatoes, beans)
saffron rice
cream cheese

———

stuffed cabbage
eggs on toast
cheese

———

Bohemian ratatouille
cheese quiche
peaches with wine

———

cabbage salad (with light cream dressing)
courgette with parsley
brie or camembert

tomato soup
1 soft boiled egg
salad of French beans
cheese

---

lasagna with herbs
stuffed mushrooms
orange mousse

What is so special about these menus?

— They ban fruit during meals.
— Separate, as much as possible, the foods rich in carbo-hydrates (starches) and food rich in proteins (meat).
— Provide, for each member of the family, ALL the necessary nutritious foods needed EACH DAY.

Only the person who WANTS TO or HAS TO slim, must reduce his dose of starches and sugars, as described in chapters IX and X.

Some exceptions can be made, but your « good sense » will tell you to « STOP » soon enough if you tend to overdo it.

One last thing about soups: you can have 1 cup, if you have to, but leave it mostly to the others. You, yourself should choose a bowl of clear broth to be drunk in the morning whilst having breakfast.

At the end of this book you'll find some new recipes, guaranteed to be light and delicious.

But first, we would like, together with you, to talk about and look for, ways to accept, and especially continue, without difficulty, the changes that will have to occur in your everyday life and nourishment. Because all this connects together - and is known as a BALANCE.

Previously we have seen how to follow an «ANTI-FAT» method without causing disorder in our family life.

We have learned that it is important to have our meals in peace and quiet.

It also is important to observe a certain method and strictness WHILE drawing up menus and shopping lists.

All this will become much more easy, once we are able to maintain this wonderful BALANCE between our body and our mind, a BALANCE which makes everything look more simple.

In order to come to this, you'll find following some easy reasonable ideas, helpful.

They are not RECIPES, (let's reserve this word for cooking), but only starters for a « BETTER - BEING » - an inner peace, a JOY OF LIVING, those being your best aids.

SECOND PART

LIVE IN PEACE
WITH YOURSELF

CHAPTER XVI

FRESHEN UP YOUR THOUGHTS

What are our most common thoughts during a day?

— I don't have time... I will be too late for the office
— The children are insufferable and ungrateful
— I've spent too much money this week
— My husband (or wife) has said some very disagreable things to me this morning
— I'm tired, my back hurts
— I'm sure I've forgotten something... but what?
— My colleague (or neighbour) makes me annoyed with her moans and groans
— They broke in to the appartment next to us, we are not safe anymore.
— My husband doesn't understand that I need to be ALONE once in a while
— I gained 5 pounds recently
— Father is ill... let's hope...
— I still have all this ironing to do
— My wife doesn't care for me anymore
— I've had it!
  etc.

Serious or futile, passing or obsessing, these preocupations fill your mind all day long.

117

They maintain a permanent tension, a never ending anxiety. You can't relax anymore, or cease this internal merry-go-round of harmful thoughts that haunt your head.

All this has its influence upon your body, especially on your nervous-and lymphatic systems, which are responsible for your entire well-being.

Without quoting any scientific explanations, that aren't ours anyhow, let's say that PEACE OF MIND is followed by PEACE OF THE BODY, which is an indispensable condition for the HARMONY we seek.

« But » you will say, « I can't prevent these endless thoughts of fear, anger or discouragement from possessing my mind... and anyway, when I look around, everybody seems to be nervous or worried! How do you expect me to be at PEACE »? There again, with the risk of repeating ourselves we can't stress enough the importance to be given to the *attitude* and necessary PRESENCE of both Father and Mother, where it concerns affections, surroundings, the atmosphere of a family. Everybody knows that the others will become more like your mirror.

They automatically return your grins as well as your smiles. There is no doubt about it that the more you show a friendly face and calm eyes, the more the atmosphere around you will become one of happiness and relaxation.

How to achieve this relative calmness, and why not, a serene and sincere peace of mind?

Well, just REPLACING, WHENEVER POSSIBLE, EACH AND EVERY NEGATIVE THOUGHT, by a POSITIVE ONE.

You should start this small internal gym during nights, when you are in bed, surrounded by darkness and quiet.

From the moment a NEGATIVE thought enters your mind (deception, resentment, jealousy, fear) say NO to it. And at the same time try to direct your thoughts to more agreable things (your child's smile, a present, a vacation plan, a happy memory) Just any thought of happiness or hope, that will replace the one that hurts you.

We have known someone, a person, who, when she started to feel exhausted, discouraged and on the edge of a nervous breakdown, started imagining herself entering a shopping center and taking WHATEVER SHE LIKED.

After a certain while, having carefully chosen and duly examined every detail: dresses, perfumes, furs, furniture, jewelry, shoes, and several other items, she wondered how to take all this home. This idea made her feel happy and she noticed that she was not feeling sad anymore. Sometimes she even fell asleep before having completed her « Raid ». So then choose your « substitute ideas » for when you are feeling distressed or exasperated.

Should you need something very spectacular to take your mind off those glum ideas, picture yourself making a movie, winning a T.V. quiz, wandering through Mexico or Japan, checking into one of those palaces in Acapulco, having a fabulous romance on a desert island... All this with the necessary details, of course, so it may last as long as possible.

The important thing to do, is to chase away the black ideas and those strains which exhaust you, and To Replace them, even by extravagant ideas, why not? If necessary?

Why? Because by acting this way, you will, little by little, come to control your thoughts, reduce your worries to their Real importance... Because, in fact, most ot the time your problems aren't that important at all, and mostly being in a good mood and confidence takes care of everything.

When you are having problems (who isn't), try to resolve them as quickly as possible, with courage and good sense. But certainly DON'T THINK OF THEM OVER AND OVER AGAIN. It's useless and depressing!

119

CHAPTER XVII

TECHNIQUE FOR «SUBSTITUTES» AND CONTROL OF IDEAS

Do you have frightening thoughts?

In your mind you must think again of something that happened in your life, that made you bold and resourceful. If necessary, think of yourself accomplishing some dangerous exploit.

A grudge against someone who has hurt you?

Remember the time you were not very polite, or dishonest, it will make you more indulgent. Imagine seeing yourself living in peace with that particular person. Or, when this is really impossible, FORGET ABOUT IT.

Problems with your marriage?

Remember the moments of happiness, the solidarity, the understanding, and all the true qualities of your partner. Imagine yourself living a beautiful love scene in the movies... it will help you.

Apprehension for the future?

Think of the difficulties our ancestors had, of their poor and monotonous food, of their primitive houses, and tell yourself that we are living in a time of tremendous progress, that will become even more important as time goes by. Imagine standing in front of an open window and looking out to an exciting future.

Are your spirits low   tired of living?

Fix your mind on things of beauty and tranquility: flowers in a meadow, sun shining through trees, animals running free, a child's smile, the colours and scents that surround us, music... All those things are free in life; take them and make them into your armoury against moral aggression and all the ugliness that frighten us sometime. There are many other reasons to be afraid and nervous...

You certainly have enough strength and imagination to find the right substitute to the right problem whenever it's necessary.

When you will have succeeded replacing in your mind all BAD by GOOD, DISCOURAGEMENT by HOPE, a big step in the right direction will have been taken.

You will be happier and more calm, and everything that surrounds you will change together with you. Little by little you will re-discover dynamic mornings and peaceful evenings.

Can you see now the LINK between your decision to lose weight and these internal exercises? When you have learnt to « control » your thoughts, you will be more « capable » to « draw up » your shopping list and menus, to « control » by mere sight, the quantity of food you will have to eat, and to « accept » with a smile, the very small privations which are necessary... All this you can do by yourself, without the help of psychotherapy, or hypnosis, without needing anybody, just in the serene tranquillity of your room.

Because, once again, in this matter, IT-S YOU who decides about everything!

CHAPTER XVIII

ASK YOUR BODY

Its our ideas, and thoughts, that control our actions. In the previous chapter we have seen how you can come to control your thoughts and replace your thoughts of fear and incapacity by thoughts of happiness and peace.

In the same way you can point your thoughts to achieving a GOAL: obtain peace at home, succeed at work, and of course, because this is what we are trying to do now: BECOME SUPPLE AND DYNAMIC AGAIN, LIKE BEFORE.

To encourage this thought, and make it more positive, we suggested you hang up your favorite picture of yourself. Looking at it each morning, you will imprint it in your mind and remember it whenever you want.

And as a wise Hindu once said:

« You can do anything, if you REALLY want to ».

« A man becomes what he thinks » which means that you can change if you Want to. « But then » you'll answer me « it won't be enough just to say to myself: « I am thirty, and I'm slim » and have it accomplished by the next day »!

Of course not! Neither I, nor You are magicians.

But if you can come to really set this idea in your mind. IT WILL HELP YOU WITHOUT YOU NOTICING IT, and everything that you will do IN THIS WAY you'll benefit from.

First thing in the morning you can start this dialogue with your body; in order to impose your will.

Talk to it. Sure. While waking up, say to it: « To-day you're going to move a little more, and breathe better.

— To start with, throw back sheets and blankets and STRETCH YOURSELF for about five minutes, breathing through your nose, and breathe out deeply. Your muscles will feel « good » at once.

— After having been to the toilet and getting dressed: do some simple FLEXABILITY exercises:

1) Standing up, arms and legs spread, turn your body quickly twice to the right, twice to the left.

2) Feet together, arms stretched before you, bend your knees keeping them together. Do this twice.

3) Standing up, feet joined together, lift one leg, bend the knee to a right angle, and, with the point of your foot, make circles. (Twice for each leg).

4) Standing up, feet joined, arms above your head, bend slowly forwards without bending your knees (twice) If you can't reach beyond your knees the first time, don't worry, You will do better each day and soon you'll be able to touch your feet.

5) Lie down on your back, lift your legs vertically, and cycle a dozen times. Then lower your legs slowly. Stay like this for a while, well stretched and breath slowly.

THAT'S ALL! and it will only take you five minutes.

CHAPTER XIX

DURING YOUR DAILY ACTIVITIES

The rest of the day is different for everyone. Some people work in a well determined place, restricted and small, others live in the middle of noise and people, commute to shopping centers and social centers, others again stay home and tend their household.

That's why, in each case, the movements of the body will be differently suited.

Working outside the home (Office, factory, shop, etc.)

1) Take the time to walk a little, either to take the bus or subway, or by getting off the bus a bit sooner, walking the rest of the way. Same thing when you return, if you have the time.

   Walk quickly, erectly, breathing deeply.

2) Whatever may be the position required for your work, CHANGE IT several times a day if possible:

— stand up and take some big steps, if you are working sitting-down.

— relax, arms on the table, arch your back, relax your legs, if you have to stand up for longer periods (sales assistant). Swing each leg several times backwards and forewards, without strain, while being supported by your fore-arms.

131

You stay at home

1) Do your shopping in the morning (see chapter: Shopping). You will have the benefit of fresh air, less people and less traffic.

2) Each time you think about it, and during your household-work, « exaggerate » your arm and leg movements AS IF YOU WERE DANCING.

3) Always open wide the windows of the room you're working in. Oxygen helps to diminish fat.

4) Do your PERSONAL FITNESS EXERCISES.
It's not necessary to take a course or to join a club, nor to force yourself into doing some difficult or painful exercises.
Trust your body and do some INSTINCTIVE movements. If possible, put on a record, or a tape with some rythmic music (Marche-Polka Quadrille) and, *alone, at home,* in front of the open window, MOVE YOUR BODY TO THE RHYTHM OF THE MUSIC.
Move your arms and legs rhythmically as you like.
The most important thing is to do movements, that OPEN WIDE the arms, straighten the chest, loosen up the pelvis. Do them to the rhythm of a typical Basque dance or the « Parisian Life » from Offenbach, and you'll see how easy they are.

5) Finally, if you want to, do some walking, cycling or swimming during your free time.

CHAPTER XX

INTERNAL MASSAGES

If performed by a real specialist, the usual massage can contribute to reduce local amounts of fat. But not everybody is able to call in the help of a good physiotherapist.

Can we massage ourselves? No, self-massage is difficult and dangerous. Difficult, because most parts of our body, which come into consideration for massage, are difficult to reach (loins, thighs, buttocks, back, etc...).

Dangerous, because a too severe massage, or rubbing in the wrong direction, can cause severe damage to the already, by fat incrusted, weakened tissues. But, if you want to try to reduce small fat concentrations by yourself, we are able to give you two EASY AND SAFE methods:

1. *The light touch by hand*
2. *Internal massage.*

The light hand strokes work with the magnetism of the hand and the reaction to it, of small muscles just under the skin.

How to proceed?

a) Rub vigorously the palms of your hands, for about two minutes, against each other. They will become hot.

b) Put them on that particular part of your body that you want to reduce. Let the warmth penetrate.

c) Your palms, slightly touching the skin, make circular movements. Goose-bumps, will be the reaction. You can do this several successive times, always after having duly rubbed your hands.

INTERNAL MASSAGE

Its origins can be bound in oriental methods, but can be perfectly adapted to our occidental morphology and temperature. Which cannot be said about several difficult and dangerous, yoga postures.

First exercise:

— Lying down on your back, (heels, thighs, shoulders and neck touching the floor) breathe deeply through your nose, while hollowing your belly. Your bust will enlarge and seem to weigh on the floor. QUICKLY, while holding your breath, stick out and hollow two or three times, your belly. Then slowly, breathe out through your mouth, relaxing the abdomen.

Second Exercise:

— Standing up, feet joined together, stretch your arms in front of you, hands open, palms facing down.
Breathe deeply (always through the nose), Then, while breathing out slowly, bend your knees as if you were to sit on your heels, and put your belly on your thighs.
Staying like this, breathe slowly two or three times, while tightening and relaxing your belly. Next you can do the

same exercise, while standing on your toes, which is even excellent for your circulation.

These massages, not only strenghten the abdominal muscles, but also help digestion, assimilation, and elimination of wastes.

And therefore, as it was for the relaxation by music, it's up to you to choose the right moment.

CHAPTER XXI

YOUR FREE-TIME

During week-ends families come together, and several activities take place.

Unfortunately, life in our big cities drives people to escape to the country or beaches. We say « unfortunately », because, this desire, understandable and excellent, makes thousands of people climb into fast cars, drive through miles of heavy traffic on dangerous roads for just a few hours of relaxation and fresh air, and repeat this every week.

It's the sin of the century and nobody can do anything about it. Holidays are almost the same for everyone, REAL country is further and further away, so, inevitably we all go to the same place at the same time.

« What shall we do »? Never go on vacation again? Of course not!

Let the big cities empty themselves every week-end, and hope that the one-day traveller finds some time to relax and breathe fresh air.

A few hours in nature, or at the beach, may compensate for this dangerous trip that made them tired, and nervous.

But, nearby small towns and villages, there are always wooods, river banks, hills, even sometimes pools and recreation-grounds. If you have the chance to live in one of these, humanly kind, places, take your family out in the fresh air during free week-ends.

It there is only the countryside or Woodlands in your neighbourhood, you can, without tiring yourself, use your muscles to walk, to row, to catch branches while stretching yourself, to crawl on your hands and knees, jump a brook, climb rocks, throw pebbles, swim...

These are NATURAL MOVEMENTS, your body is made to do them. Give it the joy of trying it without strain. Don't be embarrassed, even if at first your movements are slow and clumsy. Little by little you'll become more re-assured and capable.

You will ENJOY playing Jane or Tarzan!

Next time you go to the country, try it. There is no doubt about it, you will surely come to like it. In these games, that may seem childish to you, you will find, not only a great physical well-being and firm muscles, but more important, an ENJOYMENT OF LIFE may be lost a long time ago.

CHAPTER XXII

YOU HAVE OTHER ALLIES

As we just saw, you must use your body and mind to the utmost, if you want to achieve your goal.

But, at the same time, you must use your *SURROUN-DINGS:* the air, the sun, the water, the minerals, the plants... they are your friends, your helpers.

THE AIR

The purer it is, the richer it is in oxygen, the more it helps you to burn up the wastes of your organism.

As much as possible, let the fresh air into your house, your office, walk amidst trees (parks, squares, forests) in the early morning, breathing deeply.

BREATHE through the nose and breathe out through the mouth. If you have the courage to, do this exercise once or twice a day:

— standing up, feet slightly apart, look straight in front of you, chin forward, and join your hands behind the lower part of your back. Breathe, while swelling your lungs and, at the same time, open wide your hands from behind your back.

Then, while breathing out slowly, bring back your hands above your head making a circle at each side of your body, until your hands are back in front of your thighs.

Quickly, join your hands again behind your back and do it again (3 times).

Also « air » your body, because it is good that is should « bathe » in the air. Do you know the Chinese call the skin the « third lung »?

Wear loose clothing; of a light fibre, and when possible (climate permitting), leave your arms and legs bare and let the air caress them.

THE SUN

For a long time the sun was considered as a GOD. And this veneration is not so far off when you see how some roast their bodies on the beach.

But, as everybody knows, if sun and light are healthy, we must use them with moderation. Let the sun shine freely into your house. It makes everything more beautiful, brings light, warmth and joy.

Let it surround your body, warm your skin and joints, but don't over-do it.

But YOU, you are fragile. Your furniture and carpets, suffer from the intense warmth of a summer sun and crack or fade, but they are not vulnerable as you are.

YOU may be in the sun for only SMALL PERIODS AT A TIME and at certain times of the day only. During « the best of the day » as the peasants from the Midi would say. This means during mornings and evenings. Then you can benefit from the indirect sun rays (ultra violet) which are very healthy.

Stay out of the sun during the middle of the day. The suns rays shine directly on you (infra red) and burn and dehydrate.

Referring to the real hour of the sun (and not to the official one) you must know that you can sun bathe, without any danger, between 8 a.m. and 10 a.m. and between 4 p.m. and 6 p.m.

Each year doctors repeat this, but, the urge to « get a quick tan » is stronger and so each year the same, accidents happen (congestive pulmonary and cutaneous). You, who are sensible, expect the sun not only to give you a nice tan, but also to increase your blood flow, make you *perspire,* and help you *eliminate* toxins that poison your body and retain unsightly fat. In fact, you want it to *renew* your *energy*.

WATER

It constitutes a major part of our body, covers more than half of the entire world as a liquid or as ice, surrounds us in the atmosphere as mist or clouds. It means health, life, balance.

There have been, and there still are, long discussions about the quality of water. Certainly, it is not advisable to use impure water because not even the complex chemical processes of our bodies are able to eliminate entirely germs or other toxic elements contained in such water. That's why in town, where water is provided for consumption, it is purified through several processes.

But as regards so called « mineral waters », because of their mineral salts obtained while flowing through different types of soil, they still have all their qualities.

You can drink all of them (provided they are non-gaseous). Drink whenever you're thirsty, but *change* your brand from time to time.

147

Mostly, we will talk about water we can bathe in and which can bring a considerable help to the elimination of superfluous fat.

Sea-Baths are excellent, because they stand for physical exercises; extra oxygen and a sun-bath.

But salt water, although in has several tonic qualities, isn't a great help as regards waste elimination through the skin.

Whereas at home, we can pour into our 37° bath several products, or plant extracts which help us to slim:
— bath with Ivy leaves
— bath with seaweed

You can buy these articles in every chemist or shop where they sell natural products, and at a reasonable price.

PLANTS

The efficiency of plants doesn't need to be proven anymore. Little by little they are used again by homeopathic doctors. Flowers, twigs, leaves and roots are now to be found again at chemist's and a few remaining herbalists.

You must not expect a plant to make you lose weight at once, results will come slowly and progressively. It will be more like an addition to well balanced eating habits, that we will recommend some good herb infusions here.

It is best to let the herbs *boil* for about ten minutes or even fifteen min. So they become more active. If you take herb infusions, have them regularly, which means: one or two cups a day during at least ten days.

Stop for one week, then start again.

Of course, you are not to sweeten your infusions, except those you would drink before going to bed (½ lump of sugar only), but perfume them with some lemon drops or orange blossom water.

These are especially recommended to you:
— the catkin of the hazel
— the maize beard
— the meadowsweet
— husks of French beans
— birch tree leaves
— rosemary
— valerian
— couch grass
— fennel leaves.

IMPORTANT: Don't mix the plants. Choose the one whose taste you prefer and use it separately. Or else, use several herbs but only for ten days each.

MINERALS

They are everywhere, around us, and in us. Rocks contain minerals, the earth does, they can be dissolved in water; but plants, animals and men search for them, absorb them, live on them.

But we won't make their inventory here, as there are too many of them. Some of them can only be found in our body in extremely small amounts.

But you know most of them:
calcium, phosphorus, sodium, iron, magnesium, sulphur, potassium...

You know that serious troubles can occur if your body lacks one of them, and your doctor will have to prescribe medication containing them.

That's why we don't recommend any extreme diet which could result in diminishing the amount of mineral salts you get.

We only suggest a REDUCTION of fats, starches and sugars, and especially a DIMINISHING OF EATEN QUANTITIES by the PLATE system.

The eating habits we would like to see you adopt don't include ANY TOTAL BAN. Which means, that you will find all necessary minerals your body needs.

PRINCIPAL SOURCES OF THE ESSENTIAL MINERALS

Calcium: for YOU it will be mostly found in soft cheeses, onion, fish, cabbage, fresh fruit, yoghurt.

Phosphorus: in liver, eggs, fish, potatoes, parsley, cabbage, spinach, French beans.

Sodium: It must be present, in small quantities, in your meals. As cheese and meat already contain a large quantity of it, it is not necessary to put too much salt on your food. Also try to omit oversalted products, such as commercially cooked foods and canned food...

Iron: is to be found in: meat, fish, as well as in spinach, cabbage and poultry.

Magnesium: is found in every vegetable, but in small quantities. Wholemeal bread contains some. From time to time you can eat a small slice of it.

Sulphur: Exists in protein aliments: meat, fish, eggs, peas, wheat, milk, as well as in: apples, grape-fruit. But it is practically non-existent in canned food.

Potassium: You will find it in fresh fruit and vegetables (raw or slightly cooked), cabbage, baby peas, carrots, salad, tomatoes, celery, in pears, avocado, in skimmed milk and raw meat.

Of course, sometimes large amounts of these minerals can be found in cereals, wholemeal flour and oily fish, but as those are exactly the products you are to avoid, you must find them in those foods that are permitted to you.

Together with you, we have tried to cover the entire problem in order to reassure and convince you. If you want to slim, you must decide this calmly, still living well and eating enough in order to avoid any physical disorder.

YOUR SENSES

Senses which promote nutrition, must be well-developed in order to provide, first, a reasonable appetite, then a good stimulation of digestive juices, finally, a feeling of well-being which is excellent for perfect assimilation.

First of all we shall mention TASTE, which unfortunately today is debased from early childhood on by ready made « standard » foods, almost all prepared and sweetened in the same fashion, and given to all babies and young children alike, whatever their personal *taste*. It should be good, for their future taste preferences, to let babies eat some of the adult's soup. If they like it, let them chew a small piece of cheese omelet or swallow a spoon-full of tomato sauce. Later, from time to time, children should be allowed to choose themselves what they would like to have for their breakfast or tea-time without always giving them the same things to eat, things which are mostly *too sweet*.

If you still are lucky enough to *taste* what you're eating, you can benefit most from each bite by CHEWING THOROUGHLY.

A fresh radish, a sun-ripened tomato, a bite of a juicily roasted piece of chicken, a small piece of fresh gruyere, will then have a sublime flavour in your mouth, that you can keep longer. Yes, by chewing and mixing foods, you can still free and amplify flavours. Once the food is swallowed, you won't taste a thing anymore.

So chew as long as possible. This way, YOU WILL SWALLOW LESS QUICKLY, and therefore EAT LESS.

SMELL

SMELL is the right hand man of taste. He prepares the mouth's work and starts the formation of saliva, which contains ptyoline. This enzyme begins the transformation of starch. As this is the major provider of fat, you can understand how important this transformation in the mouth is.

So, cultivate your sense of SMELL. Don't let it become dull in a stuffy room or through superficial respiration.

Air yourself, breathe THROUGH THE NOSE and try to discover the origin of surrounding aromas (even the disagreable ones): trees, grass, leather, cloth, plants, fruits, cheeses, wood, etc...

Finally SIGHT has its part to play exciting all the other senses.

Now, you see the importance of a nicely laid table, appealing colours and presentation of well prepared dishes?

Technicians of industrial food alimentation know this very well. That's why they use artificial colours to make their products look better.

But you, you prefer natural colours, and the real scent of fresh food as they are sold to us in our local market.

It's in order to satisfy and amplify these three, so very important, senses, that it is a necessity to change menus as much as possible.

Something new, a small original detail, soft but sweet-smelling spices are then very advisable.

SEE - SMELL - TASTE these words contain all the « Know How » there is, in the art of eating.

CHAPTER XXIII

CONCLUSION

In what we've just seen, we again found the link between mind and body. This link will help you to solve, without great difficulty, the dietetical problem that worries you.

Just as you can ORDER your legs to move, your lungs to breathe deeply, so you can order your eyes to estimate the quantity of food to eat during meals.

This way, you will have the impression of REALLY being the SOLE MASTER of whatever concerns your body.

Now, you will understand, why, starting at the beginning of this book, we have said:

IT'S YOU WHO DECIDES EVERYTHING.

THIRD PART

LIGHT FAMILY
RECIPES
TO HELP YOU SLIM

OVER FORTY CALORY-FREE RECIPES

(recipes for four persons)

VEGETABLES: Stuffed tomatoes
Salad à la Chinoise
Salad Provençale
In the oven: courgettes - spinach -
aubergines - cauliflower
Leek quiche
Croquette

MEATS: Roasted veal with carrots
Kidneys
Pork with cabbage
Beef and onions
Skewers

FISH: Fresh cod with vegetables
Fried fillets
Gilthead baked in the oven
Sardines with spinach
Burbot with saffron

POULTRY:	Turkey fillets
	Fried chicken with tomatoes
	Guinea-fowl with cabbage
RABBIT:	Rabbit with mustard
EGGS:	Soft boiled egg
	Omelet, potatoes, mushrooms
	Mimosa eggs and white cheese
	Eggs and tomatoes
	Eggs au Gratin
FIRST COURSE: (warm)	Toasted cheese sandwich
	Mild vegetable salad
	Tomatoes à la Brésilienne
FIRST COURSE: (cold)	Ham roll
	Artichoke bottoms with sauce
DESSERT:	Pudding in small quantity
	Stewed fruit in wine and cinnamon
	Apple tart
LEFT-OVERS:	Shell: of meat or fish
	Mixed salad
	« Surprise » omelet
SOLE MEAL:	Calorie free sauerkraut
A LA CARTE:	Beef broth with vegetables
	Garlic sauce
FOR THOSE WHO Are in a hurry:	Carnival salad
	Escalope with lemon
	Beef Meat-loaf
	Braised courgette
	Mixed fruit mousse

VEGETABLES

STUFFED TOMATOES

— Cut them in half, remove the seeds, hollow a little. Sprinkle the bottom with some lemon juice.

Stuffing: mix, or mince, one stick of celery, two carrots, and two egg whites (of hard boiled eggs - duly minced). Dress with some olive oil and a few drops of wine vinegar. Stuff the tomatoes and decorate with a black olive.

SALAD A LA CHINOISE

Cut the raw vegetables into thin strips: two carrots, one small heart of a white cabbage, one small pepper, one chicory. A few parts of a cauliflower cut into small pieces.

Put all this in a salad bowl, add some soya shoots, then the dressing.

Dressing: Three spoonfuls of maize oil.

juice of half a lemon
basil or chervil leaves cut very thinly.
Decorate with some shrimps.

163

SALAD PROVENCE STYLE

Serve on individual *dessert* plates.

— Prepare a bed of peeled tomatoes, seeds taken out, and crushed, dressed with a spoonful of olive oil and a little lemon juice.

On this bed you put some thin rings of green pepper, young onion and hard boiled egg. Sprinkle with bits of tuna-fish (fresh and well colored) and chopped parsley.

IMPORTANT: Don't put salt into your sauces. Add only a little pepper, and put the salt-cellar on the table for the others.

GRATINS courgettes, spinach, aubergines, cauliflower
(cooked in the oven)

The principles of these Gratins are all the same, but each vegetable is prepared differently.

— *Courgettes:* are washed, brushed, cut into slices and cooked in boiling water for about ten minutes.

Aubergines: are peeled, cut into slices, left for one hour slightly sprinkled with salt in order to remove the bitterness. Then rinsed in a strainer, dried with a cloth and cooked in boiling water for about fifteen minutes.

Spinach: carefully washed, is boiled in water for fifteen minutes. Squeeze it well in order to remove all the remaining water.

Cauliflower: will be parted into small bunches, washed in water and vinegar, dipped into hot water before also being cooked for about fifteen minutes.

These vegetables: once half cooked, are put into the mixer, and then depending on your preference roughly or finely chopped. If you prefer them mashed, mix them up longer.

Gratin itself: Prepare separately:

— one well beaten egg
— 20 gms. grated gruyere cheese
— one cup of white fat free cheese
— one cup of skimmed milk
— one spoonful of fine flour or Maïzena
— garlic and chopped parsley
— juice of one lemon
— some grated bread-crumbs.

Pour a spoonful of Sunflower oil in an iron pan, with thick bottom. Once the oil is heated, put in the minced, or mashed, vegetables. While stirring, let it cook for 5 minutes, then lower the temperature. Add a little salt, pepper and the parsley. Stir some more and add the white cheese.

When everything is well mixed-up, sprinkle the spoonful of flour on top of it, stir again throughly in order to incorporate it well, add the milk, and keep on stirring.

When it has become a puree, and while stirring gently, add the whipped egg diluted in some cold water, the grated gruyere and finally the lemon juice.

Pour everything into an oven proof dish, sprinkle with grated bread-crumbs and let it brown in the oven.

Note: These (light and nourishing) gratins, can be served in the evenings together with a first course, but they must not be eaten with meat.

LEEK QUICHE

The unsweetened piecrust shell is prepared with sunflower oil instead of butter and without the addition of eggs.

You need: 4 leeks
1 jar of skimmed yoghurt
2 beaten eggs
pepper, grated nutmeg.

Wash the leek, cut it into thin slivers. Let it simmer for about 10 minutes in boiling water.

Drain it, then let it stew for about ½ hour in a Tefal pan, without any fat added.

In a salad bowl, mix the slightly chilled leek with some yoghurt, the 2 beaten eggs and the dressing.

Cover the bottom of a slightly oiled, shallow baking dish, with piecrust, pour your mixture over it and bake it a moderately warm oven (for about ½ hour).

POTATO CROQUETTES

Boil 4 potatoes in water with a stick of celery. Mash them, add 25 gms. of grated gruyere cheese.
Let it cool.

Shape the mixture into balls and roll them into the flour. When they're well covered in flour, brown them on both sides in a pan with a small amount of hot Sunflower oil.

Note: This dish should be served with green vegetables and salad - but not meat.

MEATS

VEAL ROAST WITH CARROTS

± 2 pounds Veal- (not banded with fat)
1¼ lb. of sliced carrots
12 peeled shallots.

In a pan, containing a tablespoon of sunflower oil, brown the meat on all sides. Use a moderate heat and make sure to turn round your meat frequently so it browns on all sides. Add some salt and pepper.

Once the meat is brown add the carrots and shallots. Turn them 2 or 3 times, add 1 or 2 cups of water to almost cover the vegetables. Cover the pot; leaving space for steam to escape.

Cook over a low heat for I hour. Add some water, now and then, if necessary. Once the meat is tender, pan-juices should be reduced to half.

In order to see if your meat is tender, prick it with a fork. If juices are white, your veal is ready. The carrots should also be ready by now Serve meat and vegetables separately.

Sauce should be served in a sauce-boat (for your guests *only*).

For the children give them a little a more butter with it (children usually don't like carrots).

KIDNEYS

— I veal kidney rinsed in water (some lemon juice added), remove the fat, cut into fine slices.

— 4 mushrooms de Paris sliced and steamed for 10 minutes in a dry pan.

— 12 small slices of old bread.

— Put the kidneys and mushrooms in a skillet, add 1 tablespoon of sunflower oil. Simmer until the kidney slices have lost their color and the mushrooms are ready.

Pour in small crusts of bread and stir everything well.

Finally, add some lemon juice.

Serve it hot with a puree of carrots or turnips.

PORK WITH CABBAGE

— a cabbage, sliced and boiled in water with some cumin.

—   2 lb. pork roast

— 1 cup of light vegetable broth

— Brown the roast in very little oil as it will release fat while cooking. Once it is brown add a little salt and pepper, arrange the cabbage around it together with some minced garlic and crushed tomatoes.

Stir the vegetables well, cover with hot broth. Let it cook for 1 hour. By the end of the cooking there should hardly be any liquid left over.

BEEF AND ONIONS

Very easy and delicious. Grill your steaks (chuck, sirlion steak, filet mignon) and put them on a bed of thin slices of raw onions.

SKEWERS

Everything is permitted, but to obtain a consistant cooking, don't mix up meat and vegetables indiscriminately.

With meat: (lamb, veal, pork). Use thin slices of mushrooms and peppers, raw ham, and bake them for 20 minutes.

For red meat: (mutton, beef). Use onions and thin slices of courgettes and aubergines, and bake them no longer them 10 minutes.

To go with the skewers serve a puree of tomatoes (peeled, deseeded, cooked in their own juice with just a little thyme and basil added).

FISH

COD AND DICED VEGETABLES

4 cod fillets
2 turnips cut into small strips
2 carrots cut into small strips
1 Potato
1 handful of green beans cut into pieces of approx ½ in.
1 crushed tomato
Garlic and chopped parsley.

Make a bed with the tomatoes, garlic, parsley and mixed vegetables. On top of it put the fish fillets sprinkled with a glass of lemon water and a spoonful of oil. Add a little salt, pepper. Bake them in a moderately warm oven for ½ hour.

Gild-Head Fish in the oven is prepared in exactly the same way but with some more tomatoes, and aniseed.

FRIED FILLETS

In the chapter « cooking » we have already told you how to fry fish fillets IN VERY LITTLE OIL after having dusted them thoroughly with flour. Serve them with slices of lemon, potatoes and boiled carrots.

SARDINES WITH SPINACII

Rinse the sardines, remove the central bone and if possible the skin. Roll them in flour and fry them as explained previously.

First, you will have prepared your puree of minced spinach, boiled in water, mixed and thickened with some butter and a little milk.

Serve the warm sardines on a bed of spinach, without any other dressing.

BURBOT WITH SAFFRON

— 2 pounds. Burbot without bones and skin
— 2 big tomatoes, peeled and crushed
— 1 big onion cut into small slices
— 1 chopped carrot
— freshly chopped basil
— saffron.

Put the onion and carrots in a with a tablespoon of oil. Over medium heat let them brown slightly. Add the tomatoes and basil, let it cook for 10 minutes. Add the fish and a cup of lukewarm water in which you have diluted two pinches of saffron.

Over medium heat, let it cook for about ¾ of an hour.

POULTRY AND RABBIT

TURKEY FILLETS

They are cheap but just as tasty as veal escalopes, but the need a spicy dressing.
— Let them brown in a little oil, sprinkled with garlic and chopped parsley and finally add the juice of half a lemon serve with fresh young peas or green beans.

FRIED CHICKEN WITH TOMATOES

Cut your chicken into pieces. Have the wings and legs CUT IN HALF. If you fear the chicken is not enough use 2 young cocks instead.
— 4 crushed tomatoes
— 3 chopped shallots
— chopped basil (or tarragon)
— lemon juice
— Coat the chicken pieces with flour. Let them brown in a tablespoon of oil. Take them out of the cooking pot, then put in the chopped shallots, then the tomatoes and basil. Return the pieces of chicken to your pan and pour a cup: of lukewarm water SLIGHTLY SWEETE-NED, over it.

It takes 1 hour of cooking at a moderate temperature.

Add the lemon juice just before serving.

179

GUINEA-FOWL
WITH CABBAGE

Is prepared exactly the same way as Pork with Cabbage. (for those who have to reduce their consumption of fat, it is advisable *Not to eat the skin*).

RABBIT WITH MUSTARD

(is prepared without fat or cream)

— 2 pounds of rabbit
— 3 or 4 tablespoons of mustard
— ½ oz. of soft, salted butter
— ½ glass of skimmed milk
— Coat the inside and outside of the rabbit with the mustard thoroughly mixed with the butter.

Let it bake for 1 hour in a warm oven. Turn the pieces 2 or 3 times. Half-way through cooking add 1 glass lukewarm water.

Remove the rabbit from the roasting pan, and mix the dripping with ½ glass of skimmed milk. Spoon the sauce over the rabbit.

Serve with a puree of vegetables (carrots, turnips, and a few potatoes).

EGGS

EGGS EN COCOTTE

1 egg is enough. Take 2 for the children and the hungry.

— in each small oven-proof pot: put 1 spoonful of chopped ham, break the egg on top of it. Add a little grated gruyere, some pepper and I spoonful of skimmed milk. Bake for about 10 minutes in a moderate oven.

MIMOSA EGGS AND WHITE CHEESE

— 6 hard boiled eggs. Cut them in half lengthwise.
— 1 slice of ham or 1 piece chicken fillet (minced or chopped finely)
— 1 cup of soft white cheese
— lemon juice
— some strips of red pepper.

Mix together in a bowl: ham (or chopped chicken), yolks of 5 eggs, the white cheese and the lemon juice.

Arrange the halves of the hard-boiled eggs on a plate, then fill them with the mixture, decorate them with the minced egg and a strip of red pepper.

EGGS AND TOMATOES

— 8 eggs
— 6 tomatoes: peeled and throughly mashed
— parsley
— some thyme.

Let the tomatoes soften in a nonstick pan, without adding any fat. When they are half-done add the parsley and the thyme. Crack the eggs separately 2 by 2 in bowls.

Once the tomatoes are well softened, remove the thyme.

Make 4 holes in the tomato puree and pour 2 eggs in each hole, sprinkle some pepper on each egg.

Cover the pan and let the eggs set slowly.

EGGS AU GRATIN

— 6 eggs
— ¾ pt. skimmed Milk
— 1 tablespoon of flour
— 2 oz. grated gruyere
pepper and grated nutmeg.

Hard-boil the eggs, peel them, halve them lengthwise and arrange them on an oven-proof dish (yolks up).

Prepare a white sauce separately. In a casserole dissolve the flour with COLD milk, add the butter, pepper and nutmeg. Let it thicken over a moderate heat. Keep stirring, and little by little, add the grated gruyere.

Pour this sauce on the eggs and let bake in the oven for about 10 minutes.

FIRST COURSE
(warm)

DIET CROQUE MONSIEUR
(Toasted Sandwich)

— 8 thin slices of bread (white)
— 2 slices of ham (cut in 4)
— ½ oz. grated gruyere
— 1 cup of soft white cheese.

Mix separately the grated gruyere and the white cheese. Spread half of the mixture on the slices of bread. Put a piece of ham on top of it and cover with the remaining cheese.

Put a bit of cinnamon on each Croque-Monsieur and let them grill in the oven for about 10 minutes.

MILD VEGETABLE SALAD

— 1 potato
— 2 carrots
— 2 artichoke bottoms
— 3 oz. french beans or young peas
— 6 small caulifower flowerets
— 3 oz. of boiled fish (without bones and cut into cubes)
— 1 small onion and parsley chopped together.

Poach the vegetables as explained previously. Leave them to cool, cut into bite-size pieces. Mix the vegetables with the fish in a salad bowl.

Put the salad bowl in a casserole containing 2" of boiling water, for about ¼ hour.

Meanwhile make the sauce with the onion, parsley, 2 spoonfuls of olive oil, and the juice of half a lemon.

Take the salad bowl out of the boiling water, pour the dressing over the salad, mix well and serve immediately.

BRAZILIAN TOMATOES

— Take seeds out, peel and slice 6 TOMATOES.
— Slice 2 ONIONS, blanche for 5 minutes.
— 4 hard-boiled EGGS, sliced.
— 1 spoonful of OLIVE OIL.
— 1 spoonful of BROWN SUGAR.
— Salt, pinch of Paprika, breadcrumbs.

Oil an oven-proof dish and lay alternately one layer of onions, one layer of tomatoes, slices of egg. Keep some tomatoes for the top. Add the brown sugar dissolved in half a cup of water, add a little salt and a pinch of Paprika. Top with breadcrumbs.

Cook in medium oven for ¾ hour.

FIRST COURSE
(cold)

HAM ROLL

— 4 slices of thinly cut ham
— A puree of poached and finely mixed vegetables (1 courgette, 1 leek, 1 cabbage heart, 1 carrot)
— 1 cup of cooked brown rice.

Mix the vegetables and the rice, dress with salt, pepper, parsley, sunflower oil and cider vinegar.

Spread it on the ham slices, roll them up, decorate with some parsley and a strip of red pepper.

Serve cold on some lettuce leaves.

ARTICHOKE BOTTOMS WITH SAUCE

— 8 cooked artichoke bottoms
— 1 cup of cooked maize grains
— 2 chopped hard-boiled eggs
— 8 slices of tomato
— some chopped basil.

Sprinkle a little lemon juice on each artichoke bottom. Put a good spoonful of the maize and chopped eggs mixture on it. Spread it out well and sprinkle with very little sun-flower oil.

Decorate each bottom with a slice of tomato with, in the middle, some basil. Sprinkle a little lemon juice on top of it.

REMEMBER, VERY little salt on your vegetable meals.

NONE on your meat or fish meals.

But put the salt cellar on the table for THE OTHERS.

DESSERT

PUDDING

— 1 pint of milk
— 2 eggs
— 2 spoonfuls of flour
— 1 Grated rind of a small orange
— 1 Sachet of vanila sugar
— 1 teaspoon of castor sugar.

Mix the flour and cold milk. Beat the eggs well, add them to the mixture together with the sugar, vanilla sugar and the orange peel.

Cook over a moderate heat, stirring constantly until the mixture thickens, pour into small jars and let it chill.

STEWED FRUIT IN WINE AND CINNAMON

— Apples, pears, peaches, apricots, cut into pieces (if you don't like mixed fruit, use only one kind of fruit)
— 1 glass of red wine
— 4 lumps of sugar
— 1 teaspoon of cinnamon.

Put everything in a large casserole with thick bottom, let it simmer for about 20 minutes. Spoon into cups and let it chill.

Note: If you have difficulties cutting the peaches, leave them whole or cut them in quarters. In this case they should simmer for 10 more minutes.

APPLE PIE

— 3 apples, Reinettes, peeled and diced
— 1 egg
— 1 glass of milk
— 2 oz. of flour
— 1 cup of soft white cheese
— 1 tablespoon of castor sugar
— 1 teaspoon of butter.

Butter a baking dish, spread the apples in it.

Combine the flour, the egg and the sugar in a bowl. Spoon in the white cheese and dilute with the cold milk.

Spread evenly over the apples.

Bake for about 30 minutes in a moderate oven.

LEFT-OVERS

SCALLOP SHELLS

Filled with Meat or Fish

— 12 oz. of chopped left-over meat
— 2/3 pint of milk (skimmed and boiled)
— 2 spoonfuls of flour
— 2 oz. of grated gruyere
— grated bread-crumbs.

Put the minced meat in a pan, either with some gravy (if we use yesterday's roast) or some broth (if we're talking about yesterday's « Pot Au Feu »).

Add the flour, stirring briskly and slowly pour in the milk. When the ingredients are well mixed, add the grated gruyere (first remove the pan from the fire).

Pour this mixture on the coquilles St. Jacques. Sprinkle the bread-crumbs on top of them and bake in the oven for ¼ hour.

Left-Overs of fish

Do exactly the same with fish left-overs, after having carefully skinned them and taken the bones out, and chopped them in small pieces.

MIXED SALAD

Many thing can be used for a salad. Here are some ideas:

— cooked vegetables, diced cold chicken, onions
— chicory, left-overs of rice or coquilletes, walnuts
— left-overs of « pot au feu », green salad, hard boiled eggs
— left-overs of fish, tomatoes, celery, lettuce
— chopped cress, some Dutch cheese, minced cold veal.

You can try many different things, but always keep in mind:

— Not to mix meat with fish
— Not to eat too many potatoes-if they are in your salad
— To be *reasonable* with your dressing.

SURPRISE OMELET

(serves 4)

Mix a carton of yoghurt (0% fat) and 2 spoonfuls of lukewarm water in a bowl. Crack the eggs, put them in a bowl, beat well. DON'T ADD ANY SALT, as you are to add left-overs from already salted meals.

Some suggestions:

— some chicken (without skin, bones), minced, with some chive and parsley
— some spinach or courgettes with a little grated cheese
— some ratatouille
— diced bread and some ham
— cold veal, chopped together with some onions, tomato sauce
— all kinds of hard cheese leftovers (grated).

You can use your imagination and find yourself the ingredient that will give the final touch to his surprise omelet.

200

SOLE MEALS
A la carte

This is the ideal family meal. It pleases everyone, contains all necessary ingredients for proper nourishment and still leaves those, who want to eat just a little amount, the possibility of taking as much as they want.

In the following 3 recipes you will find that they contain, of course, less fat and starches than the traditional ones. See for yourself:

CALORY-FREE SAUERKRAUT

— 2 pound raw sauerkraut
— 4 Strasbourg sausages (without colouring)
— 1 bowl of vegetable broth
— 1 small chicken
— 12 oz. of smoked bacon
— 6 small potatoes
— 1 glass of white wine
— 3 juniper berry seeds.

Wash the cabbage 3 or 4 times, the last time in hot water. Drain thoroughly. Blanche in 3 pints of boiling water for about 20 minutes. Remove the cabbage and put it in a strainer.

Blanche the bacon for about 10 minutes in some water, drain and pour away the water. Pour a spoonful of sunflower or peanut oil in a big casserole and let the bacon brown. Take out the bacon and replace it with the cabbage. Let it cook for about 20 minutes then add the white wine. Let it evaporate, pour in the broth and juniper berry seeds. Cover and let it simmer slowly for 1½ hour. Then lay the bacon on top and let it cook; again in a moderate heat.

Start baking the chicken (separately and preferably in the oven) for about ½ hour. Put in the middle of the sauerkraut, together with some of its natural juices with a little broth added.

Your sauerkraut has been cooking now for about 3 hours. On top of it you can put raw potatoes and let them cook for another 30 minutes.

Just before serving stew the Strasbourg sausages.

Pour the sauerkraut onto a large plate, the carved chicken in the middle.

The sliced bacon and the sausages are put around it. Serve the potatoes separately.

BEEF BROTH WITH VEGETABLES

— 2 lb. stewing beef
— 1 lb. veal fricasee
— 3 leeks
— 3 turnips
— 4 small potatoes
— 1 lb. of carrots
— 1 small cabbage heart
— 1 onion
— 1 stick of celery
— 1 pinch of thyme.

Pour 5 pints of water in a big casserole, add all the vegetables AND SPICES (except the potatoes). Let it cook for ¼ hour, add the joint of meat. Cook again on a moderate heat removing any scum regularly. Let it cook for another 1¼ hour.

Add the potatoes. Once the potatoes are tender, the « pot au feu » is ready. Serve the meat and the vegetables but leave the broth to chill, in order to skim off the next day.

GARLIC SAUCE

— 3 oz. sunflower oil
— 1 egg (the same temp. as the oil)
— 1 clove of garlic
— 1 tablespoon of mustard
— 1 small, cooked and still warm potato.

Crush the garlic clove in a mortar, add the potato to obtain a kind of paste. Add the mustard, the egg yolk, mix it all well. Blend in the oil drop by drop, stirring briskly. When the sauce has thickened a little, increase the amount of the oil until all the oil is incorporated.

Add a little salt and according to taste, add some lemon juice if you wish.

— If you intend to prepare your garlic sauce with the mixer, put in all the ingredients at the same time as you do for a mayonnaise.

Garlic sauce is served with hard-boiled eggs, carrots, French beans, cauliflower, beetroot, cold fish, cold meat, etc...

LIGHT MEALS FOR THOSE WHO ARE IN A HURRY

CARNIVAL SALAD

On a bed of lettuce or chopped watercress arrange rings of tomatoes, cucumbers, hard boiled eggs, previously sprinkled with oil, lemon and pepper.

Decorate with some small strips of smoked salmon or raw ham, black olives, celery leaves.

ESCALOPE WITH LEMON

— 4 thin escalopes (veal or turkey)
— bread crumbs
— chopped parsley
— lemon juice.

Dip the escalopes in the bread crumbs and let them fry in a nonstick pan (a tablespoon of oil added).

When they are brown, add the chopped parsley and the lemon. Serve hot.

BEEF MEAT-LOAF

— 1 lb. of minced beef
— 1 egg
— 1 small chopped onion
— 3 spoonfuls of flour

Mix everything well in a bowl. Add very little salt, lots of pepper. Dust a board with flour, shape patties about 2 centim. thick.

Put them in a slightly oiled skillet and fry them each side (for about 10 minutes).

BRAISED COURGETTES

— 4 well washed courgettes
— garlic, parsley
— 1 glass of skimmed milk
— 1 oz. grated gruyere.

Keep the skin on, cut them in 4. Poach them in boiling water for 10 minutes. Drain. Put them in a slightly oiled skillet and let them simmer for about 10 minutes. Add the milk, cover with the grated gruyere, cover the pan and let it simmer for another 10 minutes (without stirring).

Note: Cooking must be done over a moderate heat.

MIXED FRUIT MOUSSE

— 2 pears
— 3 apricots
— 1 peach
— 2 egg whites
— 1 sachet of vanilla sugar.

Peel, take out the stones or pips, dice and puree. Add the sachet of sugar to this mixture and let it cook gently for 10 minutes in a pot, some water added, Let it chill. Spoon the beaten egg whites on top of it. Incorporate delicately. Have it cook for another 10 minutes, spoon into individual cups and put it in the fridge for 1 hour.

Note: Don't add any sugar if the fruit is ripe.

ADDITION

As we have already mentioned in Chapter XI, we will give you some « mini menus », each of them containing only very small amounts of food. These mini menus concern those who asked us about losing their first kilos rapidly. But please remember: you ARE NOT to follow this for more than 5 DAYS.

During this time, it is better to avoid physical exertion: no spring-cleaning, no bicycle or foot races, no sport whatsoever nor receptions.

We tell you again: it's only to help those who asked us about ways of losing some weight rapidly that we have written down these special diets. We for one, prefer slimming in a gentle, progressive way, adapting freely, but definitely, our nourishment.

Hereafter you'll find 5 examples of daily food rations.

You are free to classify them, mix them up or even use only 1 or 2 of them. Approximate time schedules are mentioned for each of them, but you are free to change them at your own convenience, without of course changing THE REGULARITY OF YOUR MEALS.

Day ration n° 1

7 a.m.: warm drink (slightly sweetened) — go back to be for another 10 minutes (as already mentioned) every morning.

7.30 a.m.: cup of black coffee — 1 lump of sugar — 1 toast without butter.

Noon: 2 hard boiled eggs — some salt — 2 tablespoons of spinach — 1 Orange juice.

8 p.m.: 3 oz. grilled steak — green salad with oil and lemon.

10 p.m.: 1 cup of herb infusion without sugar.

Day ration n° 2

7.30 a.m.: black coffee — toast — 1 prune.

Noon: grilled steak — 1 tomato sliced with some sunflower oil and lemon 1 stewed fruit (diced pear or apple).

8 p.m.: 1 slice of ham — 1 yoghurt with 1 teaspoon of sugar.

10 p.m.: 1 glass of cold linden tea.

Day ration n° 3

7.30 a.m. 1 cup of vegetable broth — 1 slice of bran bread — 1 slice of ham.

Noon: fish in court-bouillon — 1 poached tomato (cooked in a pot with it's own juices, salt and pepper) — 1 slice of Dutch cheese — black coffee without sugar.

8 p.m.: salad of season fruits to which you add: ½ banana in slices and 1 spoonful of soft white cheese.

10 p.m.: 1 cup of verbena tea and ½ lump of sugar.

Day ration n° 4

7.30 a.m.: 1 cup of tea without sugar — 1 rusk — 1 spoonful of compote.

Noon: 1 chicken breast — braised celery or cooked cauliflower — 1 teaspoon of butter — 1 pear (cooked without sugar).

8 p.m.: 2 hard boiled eggs — mixed corn-salad and beetroot

10 p.m.: 1 cup of a herbal drink (made from the stems of cherries).

Day ration n° 5

7.30 a.m.: 1 cup of grated carrots dressed with some sunflower oil and lemon juice — 1 slice of toasted bread.

Noon: roasted chicken leg — warm salad of French beans — 1 black coffee.

8 p.m.: 1 grilled steak — 1 potato mashed in milk.

9.30 p.m.: ½ orange.

10 p.m.: 1 cup of herb infusion slightly sugared.

The combination and alternation of the basic elements of this diet: black coffee — hard boiled eggs — meat — allows a rather quick loss of weight. During these « mini meals » you are allowed to drink a glass of lukewarm water, some wine added. If you are thirsty in the after-noon, have some water, or herb infusion without sugar.

Finally, please remember, that this method of reduced aliments may only be used in exceptional cases, and is *not to be used longer than 5 days*.

PETRILLI TIPOLITOGRAFIA LIGURE
VIA SOTTOCONVENTO 28 VENTIMIGLIA
IMPRIME EN ITALIE